# FOOD WARS

## A GUIDE TO PROTECTING KIDS FROM PROCESSED FOOD AND SUGAR

### C. R. PURZ

# FOOD WARS

## A GUIDE TO PROTECTING KIDS FROM PROCESSED FOOD AND SUGAR

Hard cover ISBN: 979-8-35096-596-4
eBook ISBN: 979-8-35096-597-1

# DEDICATED TO PHOENIX

I hope this helps guide you,
keeps you healthy and happy.

You're the most inspiring, smart,
funny, and kind kid I've ever met.

We love you so much.

# CONTENTS

# FOREWORD

The moment a child enters your world, your priorities undergo a seismic shift. Every choice you make, every habit you form, becomes a model for this new life that looks up to you, learns from you. As a father deeply invested in the well-being of my son and having lived a life committed to health and nutrition, the journey through parenthood has been both enlightening and, at times, challenging. My dedication to a healthy lifestyle has been unwavering, rooted in a belief that the quality of the food we consume directly influences the quality of our lives. It was this belief that I hoped to instill in my son from his earliest days.

However, the reality of raising a child in a world saturated with processed foods, added sugars, and refined grains presented an unforeseen challenge. As my son grew and began to explore the wide array of foods available to him, including the ubiquitous processed and junk foods, I observed firsthand the impact of these dietary choices on his mood, his physical health, and his preferences.

The changes were subtle at first: a noticeable shift in energy levels, a growing preference for sweet and salty snacks over whole, nutrient-dense foods. It wasn't long before these dietary indulgences became a more regular part of his diet, and the effects became more pronounced. His mood began to oscillate with the highs and lows of sugar rushes and crashes. His figure, once a reflection of a child's boundless energy and a balanced diet, began to tell a different story—one of lethargy and excess.

Perhaps the most concerning development was witnessing the emergence of what can only be described as an addiction to these unhealthy foods. A request for a candy bar or a bag of chips became more frequent and insistent, demonstrating the powerful grip these foods had begun to exert on him.

This personal journey—witnessing my son's struggle with the seductive allure of processed foods—has been a poignant reminder of the challenges parents face in nurturing healthy eating habits in their children. It has reinforced my belief in the importance of understanding the profound impact that diet can have on our children's physical and psychological health.

This book, which delves into the negative effects of processed foods, added sugars, and refined grains on children, is more than a collection of research and recommendations. It is a clarion call to parents, caregivers, and society at large to recognize the urgency of this issue. It is an invitation to reflect on the dietary choices we make for our children and the long-term implications of those choices.

As you turn these pages, I encourage you to consider the information presented not just as abstract concepts, but as actionable insights that can transform the health and future of our children. The journey toward healthier eating habits is not always easy, but it is undoubtedly worth it. For in shaping the dietary preferences of our children, we are shaping their health, their well-being, and their very lives.

Let this book serve as a guide, a source of support, and a beacon of hope for all of us who hold the health of our children in our hands. Together, we can turn the tide against the rising epidemic of diet-related health issues and pave the way for a healthier, brighter future for the next generation.

Sincerely,
A Father on a Mission

In the quiet hum of modern life, amid the colorful aisles of convenience, there lies a silent epidemic shaping the destiny of our children. It's a narrative veiled behind the enticing allure of processed foods and the tantalizing sweetness of sugars. But beneath the glossy packaging and saccharine promises lies a stark reality—a reality that profoundly impacts our children's hormonal balance, emotional well-being, and physical health.

The prevalence of obesity in the United States has seen significant changes over the years. For children and adolescents aged 2–19 years from 2017–2020, the obesity prevalence was 19.7 percent, affecting about 14.7 million young individuals. The breakdown by age groups shows obesity prevalence at 12.7 percent among 2- to 5-year-olds, 20.7 percent among 6- to 11-year-olds, and 22.2 percent among 12- to 19-year-olds. Notably, obesity prevalence varied among different racial and ethnic groups, with higher rates observed in Hispanic children (26.2%) and non-Hispanic Black children (24.8%) compared to non-Hispanic White (16.6%) and non-Hispanic Asian children (9.0%) (CDC).

As of the most recent data up to March 2020, the overall obesity prevalence for U.S. adults was 41.9%, marking a significant increase from 30.5% since 1999-2000. The data also highlights that severe obesity increased from 4.7% to 9.2% during the same period. These trends underscore the serious and costly health challenge posed by obesity, which is associated with an array of health issues, including heart disease, stroke, type 2 diabetes, and certain types of cancer (CDC).

More recent statistics highlight that prediabetes is also a significant concern, affecting more than a third of American adults, many of whom may not be aware of their condition. This is indicative of a broader issue tied to dietary and lifestyle factors contributing to obesity and related health conditions (EHProject).

These statistics underscore a persistent and escalating challenge in public health, emphasizing the need for comprehensive strategies to address obesity and its associated health risks across all ages and demographics in the U.S.

REF: https://pubmed.ncbi.nlm.nih.gov/30280308/
https://www.cdc.gov/obesity/data/childhood.html
https://pubmed.ncbi.nlm.nih.gov/17243492/

In these pages, we embark on a journey to unravel the intricate tapestry of how processed foods and sugars are weaving themselves into the fabric of childhood, altering the very essence of growing up. We delve into the labyrinth of hormonal disruption, where delicate balances are disrupted, and the symphony of growth and development is thrown into disarray.

Yet, it's not just the endocrine system that bears the burden. Emotions run deep, intricately entwined with every morsel consumed. We explore the tumultuous landscape of childhood emotions, where the highs and lows are no longer just a product of youthful exuberance but also the chemical aftermath of processed indulgences. And then there's the undeniable toll on the physical vessel that carries the essence of childhood dreams and aspirations. We confront the harsh realities of burgeoning waistlines, weakened immune systems, and the ominous specter of chronic diseases casting shadows far beyond their tender years.

But amidst the darkness, there is hope—a beacon guiding us towards a future where the innocence of childhood is safeguarded, where wholesome nourishment fosters not just growth but resilience, where the sweet taste of life is savored without compromise. This is a journey not just for our children but for the generations yet to come—a journey towards reclaiming the vitality and vibrancy of youth, one mindful bite at a time.

# CHAPTER 1

# Understanding Processed Foods, Refined Sugars, and Their Hidden Dangers

---

## Processed Foods: An Overview

Processed foods are items that have undergone alterations from their original natural state for various reasons, including safety, convenience, and longevity. These modifications can encompass a range of processes such as canning, freezing, refrigeration, and packaging. The spectrum of processed foods includes moderately processed items like cheeses and fresh bread to highly processed foods such as cookies, chips, microwave meals, and sugary cereals. While processing can indeed make food more accessible and extend its shelf life, it frequently introduces unhealthy ingredients like added sugars, salt, and trans fats. The convenience of processed foods comes at a cost: a study published in the *British Medical Journal* (BMJ) found that a high intake of ultra-processed foods is associated with a significantly increased risk of cardiovascular disease and mortality.

## Refined Sugars: The Sweet Culprit

Refined sugars are extracted from natural sources like sugarcane or sugar beet through a process that eliminates impurities and other components, resulting in almost pure sucrose. This refining process removes any vitamins, minerals, or fiber originally present, leaving behind a substance that provides a quick energy boost but lacks nutritional value. Refined sugars are omnipresent in a vast array of products, from obvious ones like candy and soft drinks to less apparent items like bread and tomato sauce, significantly contributing to their calorie content without enhancing nutritional quality. The consumption of refined sugars has been directly linked to numerous health problems, including obesity, type 2 diabetes, heart disease, and even certain cancers. For instance, the American Heart Association highlights that consuming high amounts of added sugars can lead to an increase in heart disease risk factors such as elevated blood pressure and inflammation.

## Added Sugars: Hidden Everywhere

Added sugars refer to sugars and syrups added to foods and beverages during their preparation or processing. Unlike the natural sugars found in whole fruits and milk, added sugars contribute extra calories without essential nutrients. The stealthiness of added sugars lies in their prevalence in a wide variety of products, not only in sweets and desserts but also in items marketed as healthy, such as granola bars, flavored yogurts, and whole-grain breakfast cereals. The ingredient labels on food packages can be misleading, with added sugars listed under numerous aliases like high-fructose corn syrup, dextrose, maltose, and sucrose, making it a challenge for consumers to identify and limit their sugar intake. The World Health Organization recommends reducing the intake of free sugars to less than 10 percent of total energy intake, further suggesting a reduction to below 5 percent (roughly 25 grams of sugar, based on an average daily energy intake of 2,000 kcal) for additional health benefits.

## Examples of Processed Foods

Processed foods encompass a wide range of products, from minimally processed to heavily processed. Here are examples across the spectrum:

- **Moderately Processed:** These foods have ingredients added for flavor and to preserve freshness.
  - Canned fish or vegetables (with added salt or preservatives)
  - Freshly made breads (with added salt and preservatives)
  - Cheese (with added salt)

- **Heavily Processed:** Often high in added sugars, fats, and salt, these foods are significantly altered from their original state.
  - Breakfast cereals and granola bars
  - Chips and snack foods
  - Frozen meals and pizzas
  - Soda and sweetened beverages

# Examples of Refined Sugars

Refined sugars are sugars that have been processed to extract the sugar from its natural source, removing fiber and other nutrients. Common examples include:

- **White Sugar:** Also known as table sugar or granulated sugar, it's the most common form of refined sugar.

- **Powdered Sugar:** Also known as confectioner's sugar, it's granulated sugar that has been finely ground and mixed with a small amount of cornstarch to prevent caking.

- **Brown Sugar:** Consists of white sugar with varying amounts of molasses added back into it, affecting its color and flavor.

# Examples of Added Sugars

Added sugars are extra sugars and syrups mixed into foods and beverages during preparation or processing or added at the table. They can be derived from refined sugars or other sweet substances. Examples include:

- **High-Fructose Corn Syrup (HFCS):** A sweetener made from corn starch that has been processed to convert some of its glucose into fructose. Commonly found in sodas, candies, and baked goods. It's also used to extend the shelf life of food and beverage products.

- **Agave Nectar:** Though marketed as a natural sweetener, agave nectar is highly processed and high in fructose. It's used in various "health food" products and beverages.

- **Maple Syrup and Honey:** While natural, they are still considered added sugars when not consumed directly from the source. Found in baked goods, yogurts, and sauces.

- **Dextrose, Fructose, Lactose, Maltose, and Sucrose:** These are various forms of sugars added to a wide array of products, from dairy products and baked goods to canned foods and sauces.

- **Molasses:** Used in baking and for sweetening foods, molasses is an added sugar when used in processed food products.

When looking at name brand items and their sugar content, it's important to remember that formulations can change, and regional differences may exist. However, as of April 2023, here are examples of popular name brand items and the approximate amount of sugar they contain per serving. Always check the most current nutritional information on the packaging or the brand's website for the most accurate details.

## Breakfast Cereals

- Kellogg's Frosted Flakes: About 12 grams of sugar per 3/4 cup (29g) serving.
- General Mills Cinnamon Toast Crunch: Around 12 grams of sugar per 3/4 cup (31g) serving.

## Soft Drinks

- Coca-Cola Classic: Contains 39 grams of sugar per 12 oz (355 ml) can.

- Pepsi: Has about 41 grams of sugar per 12 oz (355 ml) can.

## Snack Foods

- Oreo Cookies (Nabisco): 14 grams of sugar per 3 cookies (34g).
- Nutri-Grain Soft Baked Breakfast Bars (Kellogg's): Approximately 12 grams of sugar per bar (37g).

## Yogurts

- Yoplait Original Strawberry: Contains 18 grams of sugar per 6 oz (170g) serving.
- Chobani Strawberry Greek Yogurt: About 11 grams of sugar per 5.3 oz (150g) serving (note that Greek yogurt can also have naturally occurring lactose, which is a sugar).

## Condiments and Sauces

- Heinz Tomato Ketchup: Approximately 4 grams of sugar per 1 tablespoon (17g) serving.
- Sweet Baby Ray's Original Barbecue Sauce: Around 18 grams of sugar per 2 tablespoons (36g) serving.

## Beverages

- Starbucks Vanilla Latte (Grande, 16 oz): 35 grams of sugar when made with 2g% milk.
- Gatorade Thirst Quencher, Orange: 34 grams of sugar per 20 oz (591 ml) bottle.

## Frozen Desserts

- Ben & Jerry's Chocolate Chip Cookie Dough Ice Cream: Contains 28 grams of sugar per 2/3 cup (104g) serving.

- Haagen-Dazs Vanilla Ice Cream: About 21 grams of sugar per 2/3 cup (103g) serving.

Creating a hypothetical example of a child's daily diet composed of processed foods can illustrate how easily the total sugar intake can exceed recommended limits. The American Heart Association suggests that children over the age of two should consume less than 25 grams (about 6 teaspoons) of added sugars per day for a healthy heart, and children under two years old should avoid added sugars altogether.

# Example of a Child's Daily Diet with Processed Foods:

## Breakfast

- **Cereal:** 3/4 cup of Frosted Flakes with milk—Approximately 12 grams of added sugar.

- **Beverage:** 1 cup of apple juice—Approximately 24 grams of sugar (though this may come from natural sources, frequent consumption of fruit juices is often equated with added sugars due to their high sugar concentration and lack of fiber).

## Snack

- **Yogurt:** 1 container of Yoplait Original Strawberry Yogurt—18 grams of added sugar.

- **Granola Bar:** 1 Nutri-Grain Soft Baked Breakfast Bar—12 grams of added sugar.

## Lunch

- **PB&J Sandwich:** 2 tablespoons of jelly on white bread—Approximately 12 grams of added sugar (jelly/jam).

- **Beverage:** 1 box (6.75 oz) of Capri Sun Fruit Punch—About 16 grams of added sugar.

## Afternoon Snack

- **Snack Pack:** 1 package of fruit snacks/gummies—Approximately 11 grams of added sugar.

## Dinner

- **Frozen Pizza:** 2 slices of a children's favorite frozen pizza brand—Added sugars vary but let's estimate around 5 grams for sauces and dough.

- **Beverage:** 1 can (12 oz) of soda—Approximately 39 grams of added sugar.

## Dessert

- **Ice Cream:** 1/2 cup of vanilla ice cream—Approximately 14 grams of added sugar.

**Total Estimated sugar Intake:** 153 grams of sugar

# Big Food Companies' Strategies

Large food corporations employ various strategies to boost the consumption of processed foods, especially among children, who are particularly susceptible to marketing and flavor preferences. These strategies include:

- **Marketing Tactics:** Using bright packaging, appealing cartoon characters, and engaging shapes designed to capture the attention of children. Advertisements are strategically placed during children's TV programs or on digital platforms frequented by young audiences to ensure these products are highly visible.

- **The WHO called for restrictions on marketing junk food to children:** "In 2006, WHO called for national action to protect children from marketing by substantially reducing the volume and impact of the commercial promotion of junk foods.3" and: "A 2005 study found a link between junk-food advertising to children and the risk of overweight, based on data from the USA, Australia, and eight European countries. In a 1990 study in Montreal, Quebec, English-speaking families, who were exposed to children's advertising on American television channels, had more children's cereals in their homes than did French-speaking families, who only watched Quebec channels on which advertising to children was banned." https://rb.gy/0jb92t

- **Flavor Engineering:** The incorporation of flavor enhancers and a carefully calibrated mix of sugar, salt, and fat achieves a "bliss point" that makes these foods extremely appealing and difficult to resist. This engineered palatability often leads to overeating and a preference for unhealthy food choices.

- **Hidden Sugars**: By disguising sugars under various names on ingredient lists, companies make it difficult for consumers to recognize the true amount of sugar they consume. This obfuscation tactic helps companies circumvent the growing consumer demand for healthier food options.

- **Product Placement:** The strategic placement of processed foods at eye level for children in store aisles or near checkout counters encourages impulse purchases and consumption.

- **Lobbying and Regulations:** Significant resources are allocated to lobbying efforts against regulations that would limit the ability to market unhealthy foods to children or mandate clearer labeling practices. For example, food industry lobbying has been a major obstacle to the implementation of soda taxes in various regions, which aim to reduce consumption of sugary drinks.

- **Overall Food Industry Lobbying:** According to data from OpenSecrets, the food and beverage industry spent approximately $29 million on lobbying efforts in 2022 alone.

- **Specific Company Expenditures:**

  ◦ Coca-Cola Company: Spent about $8.7 million on lobbying in 2022

  ◦ PepsiCo Inc: Spent around $3.4 million on lobbying in 2022

  ◦ American Beverage Association: Spent approximately $1.5 million on lobbying in 2022

- **Soda Tax Opposition:** In Berkeley, California, the American Beverage Association spent $2.4 million campaigning against a soda tax measure in 2014.

- **Nutrition Labeling:** When the FDA proposed changes to nutrition labels in 2014, the Grocery Manufacturers Association spent $3 million lobbying against the changes.

In writing this chapter, my goal was to cast a spotlight on the complex and hazardous landscape of our current diets, heavily populated with processed foods and refined sugars. This exploration was intended not only to delineate the transformation of natural foods into their processed counterparts but also to underscore the health risks associated with this dietary shift. From the minimal processing of vegetables to the heavy alteration of snack foods, and the pervasive presence of refined and added sugars, these elements collectively contribute to the rising tide of health issues such as obesity, diabetes, and cardiovascular diseases.

It's imperative to challenge the status quo of dietary habits and the food industry's influence on consumer choices. The deceptive marketing strategies employed by large food corporations, particularly those targeting vulnerable young consumers, is a critical concern. These strategies cleverly mask the harmful content of products under the guise of fun packaging and compelling advertisements, making it increasingly challenging for individuals to make health-conscious dietary choices.

The research and insights compiled in this chapter solidified my belief in the necessity of a dietary pivot towards whole, unprocessed foods for both individual and societal well-being. I advocate for stronger regulatory measures to reign in the misleading practices of the food industry and for enhanced transparency in the labeling of food products, to empower consumers with the knowledge to make informed choices.

My call-to-action centers on a more enlightened approach to our dietary choices and a concerted effort to shift towards food practices that prioritize nutrition and health. The evidence presented is a call to reevaluate our food system and personal eating habits, advocating for a diet that embraces simplicity and nutritional integrity over convenience and allure. It is my hope that this chapter inspires readers to critically examine their own and their children's diets and to demand a food environment that nurtures, rather than compromises, our health.

# CHAPTER 2

# Unmasking the Silent Sleeper Agent:
## *The Fructose in Processed Foods*

---

The dietary landscape of modern society is increasingly dominated by processed foods, within which a silent sleeper agent—
high fructose—plays a covert yet significant role. This chapter delves
deeper into the complexities of fructose as an additive, examining its
widespread, yet often unnecessary, addition to a multitude of products and its far-reaching impact on health, particularly in children.

## The Infiltration of Fructose

Fructose naturally occurs in fruits, where it is accompanied by fiber,
vitamins, and minerals, contributing to the fruit's nutritional profile.
However, the fructose that stealthily infiltrates processed foods is a
far cry from its natural counterpart. Extracted and isolated, it becomes
a potent sweetener known as high-fructose corn syrup (HFCS).
HFCS's appeal to the food industry is multifaceted: it's cheaper than
natural sugar due to corn subsidies, it extends product shelf life,
and its intense sweetness enhances flavor, making products more
appealing to consumers.

The use of HFCS skyrocketed in the late twentieth century and is now prevalent in sodas, sweets, bread, cereals, and even less obvious products like ketchup and salad dressings. This widespread use has paralleled and arguably contributed to rising health issues globally. The CDC reports that from 1999 to 2018, the prevalence of obesity in U.S. children and adolescents aged 2 to19 years increased from 13.9 percent to 19.3 percent.

The type of fructose commonly added to foods is typically in the form of High-Fructose Corn Syrup (HFCS) as stated above but the below is further detail on types of HFCS and other forms of high fructose that are added to processed foods:

- **High-Fructose Corn Syrup (HFCS):** This is the most common form of added fructose in processed foods. It's made from corn starch and contains varying ratios of fructose to glucose. The two most common forms are:

- **HFCS 55:** Contains 55% fructose and 45% glucose. This is commonly used in soft drinks.

- **HFCS 42:** Contains 42% fructose and 58% glucose. This is often used in processed foods and baked goods.

- **Crystalline Fructose:** This is a more purified form of fructose that's nearly 100% fructose. It's sometimes used in beverages and processed foods for added sweetness.

- **Agave Nectar:** While often marketed as a natural sweetener, agave nectar is highly processed and can contain up to 90% fructose.

- **Fruit Juice Concentrates:** These are sometimes used as sweeteners and do contain fructose, though they're often marketed as more natural alternatives to HFCS.

- **Invert Sugar:** This is a mixture of glucose and fructose produced by splitting sucrose molecules. It's sometimes used in food manufacturing.

It's important to note that while fructose occurs naturally in fruits and some vegetables, the fructose added to processed foods is often in concentrated forms like HFCS, which can be consumed in much larger quantities than would be possible through whole fruits. This high concentration and volume of consumption are what contribute to health concerns associated with added fructose in the diet.

## Effects on the Body

- **Liver Overload and Fat Production:** With high-fructose intake, the liver can become overloaded and start turning fructose into fat through a process called lipogenesis. This can lead to the accumulation of liver fat, contributing to non-alcoholic fatty liver disease (NAFLD).

- **Insulin Resistance and Type 2 Diabetes:** The liver's conversion of fructose to fat can also cause an increase in the production of triglycerides. High levels of triglycerides can lead to insulin resistance, where the body's cells become less responsive to insulin. Insulin resistance is a precursor to type 2 diabetes and is associated with increased risk of cardiovascular disease.

- **Increased Uric Acid Levels:** Fructose metabolism produces uric acid as a byproduct. High levels of uric acid can lead to gout, a type of arthritis characterized by painful inflammation of the joints. Additionally, elevated uric acid levels are associated with increased blood pressure and cardiovascular risk.

- **Appetite Dysregulation:** Unlike glucose, fructose does not stimulate insulin secretion or enhance leptin production (a hormone involved in regulating hunger and energy balance). This lack of regulatory feedback can lead to increased calorie intake because the body does not receive the usual signals of satiety, potentially contributing to weight gain and obesity.

- **Gut Health and Inflammation:** Emerging research suggests that excessive fructose consumption may alter the gut microbiota, leading to increased intestinal permeability (leaky gut). This condition can allow endotoxins to enter the bloodstream, triggering inflammation and exacerbating metabolic disorders like insulin resistance and obesity.

## Physical Repercussions

The liver metabolizes fructose differently from glucose, the other main sugar found in carbohydrates. Excessive high fructose consumption can lead to an overload of the liver's metabolic capacity, resulting in increased fat production and storage—a pathway to obesity and insulin resistance. This is particularly concerning for children, whose diets are increasingly high in HFCS. Obesity is not the only concern; studies have shown a significant link between high fructose intake and the development of nonalcoholic fatty liver disease (NAFLD) in children, a condition historically associated with alcohol abuse but now emerging in pediatric populations due to dietary habits.

## Mental and Emotional Dimensions

The impact of fructose extends beyond the physical, affecting cognitive function and emotional well-being. Diets high in added sugars impair cognitive abilities, disrupt learning processes, and are linked to lower academic achievement. Furthermore, the volatility of blood sugar levels associated with high-fructose consumption can lead to mood disturbances, exacerbating conditions like anxiety and depression. This is particularly detrimental to children, for whom emotional stability is crucial for developmental and social growth.

## Pervasive Yet Unnecessary

The nutritional benefit of added high fructose in processed foods is nil; its inclusion is driven by taste, addiction, and, of course, economics rather than health. For example, fruit-flavored yogurts often contain more HFCS than fruit, misleading consumers about their health value. Such deceptive practices contribute to an environment where excessive sugar consumption is normalized, despite its clear health risks.

## Towards a Healthier Path

Combatting the ubiquity of high fructose in processed foods requires informed consumer choices and a shift in dietary habits towards whole, unprocessed foods. By choosing real fruits over fruit-flavored imitations and preparing meals from fresh ingredients, families can significantly reduce their fructose intake. Education plays a crucial role, empowering parents and children to decipher food labels and understand the long-term consequences of their dietary choices.

Here are examples of processed foods and categories where fructose, particularly as HFCS, is frequently added:

## Soft Drinks and Sweetened Beverages

- **Cola and other sodas:** Many popular soda brands use HFCS as a primary sweetener.

- **Sweetened iced teas:** Bottled or canned iced teas often contain HFCS or other fructose derivatives for sweetness.

- **Energy drinks:** In addition to caffeine, many energy drinks are high in HFCS, contributing to their sweet taste.

- **Fruit-flavored drinks:** These beverages, which may contain little to no actual fruit juice, often use HFCS as a cheap sweetener.

## Snack Foods and Sweets

- **Candy:** A wide variety of candies, including gummies, hard candies, and chocolate bars, contain HFCS.

- **Packaged snacks:** Snack foods like granola bars, flavored popcorn, and fruit snacks frequently list HFCS among their ingredients.

## Baked Goods

- **Commercially baked breads:** Some breads and buns include HFCS, contributing to a slightly sweet taste and improved shelf life.

- **Pastries and cakes:** HFCS is used in many commercially produced pastries, cakes, and cookies for sweetness and moisture retention.

## Condiments and Sauces

- **Ketchup:** HFCS is a common ingredient in many brands of ketchup, enhancing its sweetness.

- **Barbecue sauces:** Many barbecue sauces are high in HFCS, contributing to their sweet, tangy flavor profile.

- **Salad dressings:** Certain sweet or creamy salad dressings use HFCS as a sweetener.

## Dairy Products and Alternatives

- **Flavored yogurts:** Many flavored yogurts, especially those targeting children, contain HFCS or fructose as sweeteners.

- **Ice cream:** Some ice cream brands use HFCS to sweeten their products, particularly in flavors with caramel or syrup swirls.

## Breakfast Foods

- **Cereals:** Many breakfast cereals, even those marketed as healthy, can contain HFCS as a primary sweetening agent.

- **Pancake syrups:** Most commercial pancake and waffle syrups are primarily made from HFCS, with little to no real maple syrup.

It's evident that the quiet infiltration of HFCS into our diets represents a significant and underappreciated threat to public health, particularly among our youngest. This chapter has unveiled the stark contrast between the benign presence of fructose in natural fruit and its potent, isolated form as high-fructose corn syrup (HFCS) in processed foods—a form that has become all too common and carries with it serious health implications. From its contribution to the alarming rise in obesity and nonalcoholic fatty liver disease (NAFLD) among children, to its role in insulin resistance, increased uric acid levels, and the dysregulation of appetite, the evidence is clear: the impacts of fructose extend far beyond the sweet taste it imparts to our foods.

Moreover, the mental and emotional toll of high fructose consumption cannot be overstated, affecting everything from cognitive function to emotional stability in children. The pervasive use of HFCS, driven by factors of cost, taste, and addictive properties rather than nutritional value, calls for an urgent reevaluation of our dietary choices and the policies that shape our food environment.

Let this chapter serve as a call to action—not just for individuals, but for policymakers, educators, and food manufacturers—to consider the profound effects of our dietary environment and to work towards a healthier, more transparent food system.

The path forward requires a concerted effort to reduce our reliance on processed foods and to seek out whole, unprocessed alternatives. By doing so, we can begin to counteract the stealthy yet significant impact of high fructose on our health. Education and awareness are paramount; consumers must be empowered to make informed decisions about their diets, understanding the long-term health implications of excessive fructose consumption.

In moving towards a future where whole foods take precedence and informed choices are the norm, we can hope to address not just the issue of high fructose, but the broader challenges of dietary health that face our society.

# CHAPTER 3

## The Dire Consequences of Processed Foods and Sugars on Children's Health

---

The surge in consumption of processed foods and added sugars, particularly fructose, has emerged as a critical concern in the current dietary landscape, with profound implications for the health and development of children. These elements exert a significant influence on both the physical and hormonal dimensions of health, critically shaping children's growth, development, and overall well-being.

### The Alarming Physical Health Impacts

- **Obesity and Its Complications**: The stark increase in childhood obesity is one of the most visible and concerning effects of a diet laden with processed foods and added sugars. The empty calories and low nutritional content of these foods contribute to excessive weight gain, setting the stage for a lifetime battle with obesity and its associated risks, including heart disease, type 2 diabetes, and certain forms of cancer.

- **The Rise of Type 2 Diabetes in Youth**: Once a rarity in the pediatric population, type 2 diabetes now mirrors the obesity epidemic, with its incidence climbing alarmingly among children. This condition not only demands lifelong management but also increases the risk of severe complications, including organ damage and cardiovascular disease.

- **Non-Alcoholic Fatty Liver Disease (NAFLD)**: The excessive intake of fructose-rich products is a key driver behind the increasing prevalence of NAFLD among children, marking a condition where fat accumulation in the liver could lead to inflammation, scarring, and irreversible damage.

- **Dental Health Deterioration**: The pervasive sweet and acidic nature of processed foods has led to a marked increase in dental problems among children, including cavities and tooth decay, with significant consequences for their pain levels, eating habits, and speech development.

## Hormonal and Developmental Effects

- **Insulin and Leptin Resistance**: The disruption in insulin and leptin signaling, induced by excessive sugar and processed food intake, underlies a multitude of metabolic disorders. These conditions complicate the management of healthy body weight and energy balance and are increasingly documented in the pediatric population.

- **Precocious Puberty**: Emerging research indicates a disturbing link between high consumption of processed foods and sugars and the early onset of puberty. This premature development carries profound psychological and physical health implications, heightening the risk for various cancers and metabolic diseases in later life.

- **Impaired Growth and Development**: Critical nutritional deficiencies, resultant from a diet dominated by processed foods, can severely disrupt the natural production of growth hormones, essential for children's physical and cognitive development.

# Beyond Physical Health:
# The Psychological and Behavioral Fallout

- **Cognitive Decline and Academic Challenges**: Diets high in sugars and processed foods have been implicated in diminishing cognitive functions, including memory, attention, and learning abilities, which in turn, can severely impact academic achievement and future opportunities.

- **Mood Disorders and Behavioral Problems**: The erratic blood sugar fluctuations associated with high sugar intake are linked to mood instabilities, hyperactivity, and an elevated risk of mood disorders, such as depression and anxiety, complicating children's emotional regulation and social interactions.

- **Addictive Eating Patterns**: The dopamine release triggered by processed foods and sugary snacks is akin to that caused by addictive substances, fostering patterns of compulsive eating and food addiction from a young age.

# 1. Obesity

Childhood obesity is a condition where a child is significantly over the normal weight for their age and height. An example would be a ten-year-old child weighing significantly more than the average for their age group, often calculated using body mass index (BMI) percentiles. This condition can lead to various health issues, including early signs of cardiovascular disease such as elevated blood pressure and cholesterol levels.

# 2. Type 2 Diabetes

A twelve-year-old child frequently consuming high-sugar drinks and snacks develops signs of insulin resistance, such as dark patches on the skin (acanthosis nigricans) and experiences increased thirst, urination, and unexplained weight loss. A medical evaluation reveals elevated blood sugar levels, leading to a diagnosis of type 2 diabetes.

# 3. Non-Alcoholic Fatty Liver Disease (NAFLD)

An eleven-year-old who eats a diet high in fructose, primarily from sugary beverages and processed snacks, starts showing elevated liver enzymes during a routine checkup. Further examination, including an ultrasound, indicates fatty deposits in the liver, leading to a diagnosis of NAFLD despite the child not consuming alcohol.

> "Data from 2017 to 2021 shows large jumps in the incidence of nonalcoholic fatty liver disease across all ages in the nation, but the steepest increase by far is in children. For children up to age 17, the rate of diagnosis more than doubled, according to insurance claim data analyzed for The

Post by Trilliant Health." Nutritional surveys show that meals eaten by kids changed radically in a generation, going from very little ultra-processed foods in the early 1980s (they hadn't hit the market in a big way yet) to more than 67 percent in recent years. Such diets lead to hormonal changes and other stresses on our bodies."

"It creates a time bomb, and it is killing our kids," said Barry M. Popkin, a professor of nutrition at the Gillings School of Global Public Health at the University of North Carolina at Chapel Hill.

Source: *Washington Post* https://www.washingtonpost.com/health/interactive/2023/nonalcoholic-fatty-liver-disease-kids/

## 4. Dental Health Issues

A seven-year-old with a fondness for candy and soda presents with multiple dental cavities and tooth decay. The child complains of tooth pain and sensitivity to hot and cold, prompting a visit to the dentist, who identifies the need for several fillings due to extensive dental caries.

## 5. Insulin Resistance

A thirteen-year-old overweight child, with a diet rich in processed foods and lacking in physical activity, shows signs of insulin resistance, such as difficulty concentrating and fluctuating energy levels. Blood tests reveal higher than normal insulin levels, indicating the body's cells are becoming less responsive to insulin.

# 6. Early Onset of Puberty

An eight-year-old girl begins showing signs of puberty, such as breast development and the start of menstrual periods, much earlier than her peers. Her diet, high in processed foods and added sugars, is considered a contributing factor to this early maturation, leading to concerns about her physical and psychological well-being.

# 7. Growth and Development Issues

A nine-year-old boy, predominantly consuming processed foods with minimal nutritional value, shows stunted growth and delayed developmental milestones compared to his peers. Nutritional deficiencies, particularly in essential vitamins and minerals necessary for growth, are identified as a significant factor.

These examples illustrate the direct impact that a diet high in processed foods and added sugars can have on children's health, leading to serious conditions that can affect their quality of life, both immediately and in the long term.

As we wrap up chapter 3, the critical insights gathered underscore the urgent need for action against the pervasive influence of these dietary elements. The analysis presented reveals not only the alarming physical health impacts—ranging from obesity and its complications to the rise of type 2 diabetes and nonalcoholic fatty liver disease in children—but also the profound hormonal and developmental effects, including insulin and leptin resistance and the unsettling trend towards precocious puberty. The dietary patterns entrenched in our society are setting the stage for a host of health challenges that extend beyond the immediate physical ailments to encompass cognitive decline, mood disorders, and addictive eating patterns, all posing significant barriers to children's academic achievement, emotional stability, and overall well-being.

In confronting this crisis, it becomes clear that collective efforts are required to reverse the tide. This calls for a comprehensive approach that spans education, policy reform, and community support to foster environments that promote nutritional health and well-being. By prioritizing whole, nutrient-dense foods and advocating for policies that limit the prevalence of processed foods and added sugars in our children's diets, we can begin to mend the fabric of their health and secure a more promising future.

The journey towards a healthier tomorrow for our children demands vigilance, commitment, and a willingness to challenge the status quo. Let this chapter serve as a catalyst for change, inspiring individuals, families, and communities to take a stand for the health of our youngest members. Together, we can turn the tide against the dire consequences of processed foods and sugars, paving the way for a generation of children who thrive in health, happiness, and potential.

# CHAPTER 4

## Navigating the Mental and Emotional Maze: *The Role of Diet in Children's Development*

---

The dramatic increase in the consumption of processed foods, refined sugars, and fructose is not just a physical health crisis but a growing concern for the **mental and emotional** development of children. This dietary trend is casting long shadows over the cognitive growth, emotional stability, and overall mental well-being of young minds, prompting a critical evaluation of our food choices.

## The Cognitive Impact of Processed Foods

- **Nutritional Foundations for Brain Development**: The young brain's architecture, designed for rapid growth and learning, relies heavily on a steady supply of key nutrients. Omega-3 fatty acids, iron, zinc, and vitamins, pivotal for cognitive development and neural connectivity, are often missing in processed food diets. This nutritional gap can lead to noticeable deficits in memory, attention, and

problem-solving skills. The absence of these critical nutrients in diets high in processed foods can have tangible
effects on a child's cognitive development. Deficiencies
can lead to deficits in memory—both working memory and
long-term memory—reduced attention span, and diminished problem-solving skills. Over time, these cognitive
impairments can affect academic performance, social
interactions, and overall quality of life. Given the brain's
remarkable plasticity during childhood, ensuring a diet
rich in these key nutrients is paramount for fostering robust
cognitive development and neural connectivity. This nutritional investment in the early years lays the groundwork
for a lifetime of learning, adaptability, and mental health.

- **The Sugar-Cognition Paradox**: The modern diet, with its
high content of refined sugars and fructose, presents a
paradoxical challenge to the developing brains of children.
While these sugars can temporarily boost energy levels,
their overall impact on cognitive function and academic
performance is decidedly negative. This phenomenon,
known as the Sugar-Cognition Paradox, highlights the complex relationship between dietary sugars and brain function.

## Blood Glucose Fluctuations and Cognitive Function

Refined sugars and fructose lead to rapid spikes in blood glucose
levels followed by equally swift declines—a cycle that can have
immediate and adverse effects on cognitive abilities. Glucose is a
primary energy source for the brain, and while steady levels support
cognitive functions, erratic fluctuations disrupt them. After consuming sugary foods or drinks, children may experience a short-lived
increase in alertness and energy. However, this is quickly followed

by a "crash" in energy levels, characterized by fatigue, irritability, and decreased attention span. These fluctuations can impair the brain's ability to process information, store memories, and maintain concentration—all skills critical for learning.

## The Impact on Academic Performance

A growing body of research has established a link between high-sugar diets and diminished academic performance. Studies have shown that children who consume diets high in refined sugars score lower on academic assessments and display reduced cognitive capabilities compared to their peers with lower sugar intake. The reasons are multifaceted but center around the sugar-induced disruption of blood glucose stability, leading to difficulties in maintaining focus, processing information, and performing complex cognitive tasks. These challenges make it harder for children to engage fully in the learning process, ultimately affecting their academic achievements.

## The Role of Sugar in Attention and Memory

The adverse effects of high sugar consumption extend to specific cognitive domains critical for academic success, such as attention and memory. Sugar-induced blood glucose fluctuations can significantly impact a child's ability to sustain attention on tasks or activities, leading to increased distractibility and decreased productivity. Similarly, memory—both working memory and long-term memory—can be affected, making it challenging for children to retain new information and skills. These cognitive impairments can hinder not only day-to-day learning but also long-term educational outcomes.

## Addressing the Sugar-Cognition Paradox

Mitigating the negative impact of refined sugars and fructose on children's cognitive development and academic performance requires a multifaceted approach. Reducing the intake of sugary foods and beverages while promoting a balanced diet rich in whole foods can help stabilize blood glucose levels, supporting sustained energy and cognitive function throughout the day. Additionally, educating children, parents, and educators about the cognitive risks associated with high-sugar diets is crucial. By fostering an awareness of the Sugar-Cognition Paradox, stakeholders can encourage healthier eating habits that support not only physical health but also cognitive development and academic success.

The Sugar-Cognition Paradox underscores the need for a reevaluation of dietary patterns among children, emphasizing the critical role of nutrition in cognitive function and academic performance. By understanding and addressing the impacts of refined sugars and fructose, society can better support the cognitive development and educational achievements of future generations, ensuring that children have the nutritional foundation needed to reach their full potential.

# Emotional Development in the Crosshairs

- **Regulating Emotions in a Sugar-Laden World**: The ability to navigate one's emotional landscape is a fundamental aspect of development. Diets rich in processed foods destabilize blood sugar levels, leading to mood swings and irritability. This volatility can obstruct a child's journey towards effective emotional regulation, paving the way for increased frustration, sadness, and behavioral issues.

- **The Diet-Stress Connection**: Chronic reliance on unhealthy foods primes the body's stress response, heightening susceptibility to anxiety and depression. The modern diet, laden with additives and devoid of essential nutrients, can exacerbate the body's reaction to stress, leaving children less equipped to handle emotional challenges.

## Diet and Mental Health: A Troubling Link

- **A Pathway to Depression and Anxiety**: The intricate relationship between diet and mental health is gaining recognition, with poor dietary habits being linked to an increased risk of depression and anxiety among children. The absence of crucial nutrients from processed foods can disrupt neurotransmitter balance, crucial for mood regulation, heightening the risk for these conditions.

- **ADHD and Dietary Patterns**: The prevalence of ADHD symptoms, such as inattention and hyperactivity, has been observed to worsen with diets high in processed foods and sugars. Although the connection is multifaceted, dietary modifications have shown potential in alleviating these symptoms, highlighting the role of nutrition in managing ADHD.

## Towards Mental and Emotional Wellness

- **A Dietary Blueprint for Well-being**: Combatting the mental and emotional repercussions of processed food consumption necessitates a dietary overhaul. Emphasizing whole, nutrient-dense foods can nourish the brain, support emotional development, and foster mental health.

Families and educators play a pivotal role in guiding children towards healthier eating patterns, emphasizing the importance of fruits, vegetables, whole grains, and lean proteins.

- **Educational Imperatives**: Raising awareness about the profound impact of diet on mental and emotional well-being is crucial. Integrating nutrition education into curriculums and family life can empower children to make informed food choices, laying the groundwork for a lifetime of cognitive and emotional resilience.

It becomes increasingly clear that the stakes of our dietary choices reach far beyond the physical, deeply influencing the cognitive growth, emotional resilience, and mental well-being of our children. The discussion has shone a light on the complex interplay between diet and development, revealing how processed foods and high sugar intake not only compromise the nutritional foundations essential for brain growth but also pose a paradoxical threat to cognitive function and academic performance. This Sugar-Cognition Paradox, characterized by the immediate yet fleeting boost in energy followed by a sharp decline, underscores the detrimental effects of refined sugars on attention, memory, and learning capabilities.

Moreover, the emotional and mental health ramifications of such dietary patterns are profound. From the volatility in mood and emotional regulation challenges to the heightened risk of anxiety, depression, and ADHD symptoms, the evidence presented paints a troubling picture of the impact of diet on the emotional landscape and stress management capabilities of children.

Addressing these concerns requires a multifaceted strategy that extends beyond the individual to encompass families, educators, and policymakers. It involves a fundamental shift towards whole, nutrient-dense foods that support cognitive and emotional development, alongside a concerted effort to educate and empower children and their caregivers about the importance of dietary choices. This chapter serves as a call to action—to recognize and respond to the critical role that diet plays in shaping the mental and emotional fabric of our children's lives.

By prioritizing nutrition that fuels both the body and mind, we pave the way for a future where children can grow into mentally resilient and emotionally balanced individuals. This commitment to fostering nutritional well-being offers a pathway to mitigating the mental and emotional challenges faced by our youth, ensuring they have the foundation to navigate life's complexities with confidence. As we move forward, let us hold close the understanding that our food choices are not merely about sustenance but about nurturing the holistic development of our children, ensuring they thrive in every sense of the word.

# CHAPTER 5

## Navigating the Maze: *Processed Food and Sugar Addiction in Childhood*

---

The escalating consumption of processed foods and refined sugars among children is not merely a dietary concern but a harbinger of deep-seated addictive behaviors. This chapter aims to dissect the multifaceted nature of addiction to these substances, revealing how they can alter a child's behavior and potentially set a trajectory towards a lifetime of unhealthy eating habits.

## Delving into Addiction

- **Physiological Dependence**: The addictive nature of processed foods and refined sugars is intricately linked to their impact on the brain's reward system—a complex network influenced by neurotransmitters that regulate feelings of pleasure and satisfaction. Foods high in sugar, fat, and salt are particularly potent in stimulating the release of dopamine, a neurotransmitter often referred to as the "feel-good" chemical. This reaction is not unlike that triggered by addictive substances, where the consumption of these foods leads to a temporary surge in dopamine levels, providing an immediate sense of pleasure and reward.

The cycle of dependence on processed foods and sugars is fueled by the body's adaptation to these dopamine surges. Over time, the brain requires larger quantities of these foods to achieve the same level of satisfaction, creating a cycle of cravings and dependence reminiscent of substance addiction. A pivotal study published in the journal *Pediatrics* shed light on this phenomenon by demonstrating the significant dopamine release triggered by sugar intake, underscoring its addictive potential on par with certain drugs. This physiological dependency not only fosters a persistent craving for these foods but also establishes a pattern that can be difficult to interrupt.

• **Emotional Reliance**: The addiction to processed foods and refined sugars extends beyond physiological responses, enveloping an emotional dimension that compounds its complexity. For many children, these foods become a source of comfort and escape from negative emotions such as stress, loneliness, or boredom. The immediate gratification they provide can become a learned response for emotional regulation, deeply embedding sugary and processed foods into a child's coping mechanisms.

This emotional reliance on unhealthy foods for comfort is not a fleeting childhood phase; it has the potential to solidify into long-lasting behavioral patterns. As these children transition into adulthood, the emotional ties to food can persist, complicating efforts to adopt healthier eating habits.

This entrenched behavior not only poses challenges for physical health but also for emotional well-being, as it can perpetuate a cycle of guilt, shame, and continued reliance on food for emotional solace.

The intersection of physiological dependence and emotional reliance on processed foods and sugars paints a comprehensive picture of the addictive nature of these substances. It highlights the urgent need for strategies that address both the biological and emotional facets of food addiction. Interventions that encompass dietary education, emotional support, and healthier coping mechanisms are essential in breaking this cycle, offering hope for those caught in the web of food addiction.

## Cognitive Conditioning and Reward

Mental addiction begins with cognitive conditioning. The human brain is remarkably adept at forming associations between actions and rewards. When consumption of processed foods or sugars leads to pleasurable outcomes, such as a dopamine surge or emotional relief, the brain starts to associate these foods with positive experiences. Over time, this conditioning strengthens, creating powerful mental cues that trigger cravings for these foods, independent of actual hunger or physiological need.

This reward-based learning is compounded by the omnipresence of processed foods in daily life and their glorification in media and advertising. Such exposure reinforces the mental addiction, making processed foods the "go-to" solution for a variety of emotional states, from celebration to consolation.

# Habit Formation and Routine

Another key component of mental addiction is the formation of habits and routines centered around processed foods and sugars. Habits, once established, operate largely outside of conscious awareness, guiding behavior with little deliberate thought. For many, routines such as a sugary snack after school or a visit to a fast-food restaurant become ingrained parts of their daily lives. Breaking these habits requires not only an awareness of their existence but also the deliberate effort to form new, healthier routines.

# The Role of Memory and Emotional Eating

Memories of past pleasures associated with eating processed foods play a significant role in mental addiction. These memories can trigger intense cravings, especially during times of emotional vulnerability. Emotional eating, a common manifestation of food addiction, is driven by the desire to recapture the comfort and solace previously found in these foods. This cycle is self-perpetuating, as the act of seeking emotional relief through food reinforces the cognitive associations that fuel addiction.

# Behavioral Shifts

- **The Snack Cycle**: The ritual of reaching for sugary snacks or beverages can evolve from a mere habit to an essential coping mechanism, manifesting in mood swings, agitation, or distress when these foods are unavailable. Such patterns disrupt not only nutritional health but also emotional stability, promoting a reliance on food for emotional regulation.

- **Avoidance of Nutritious Foods**: The allure of processed foods often leads to a disinterest in healthier, less stimulating options. This taste preference, cultivated early, can result in nutritional gaps and a lifelong struggle to incorporate balanced meals into one's diet.

- **Secret Consumption**: As children become cognizant of the societal and familial scrutiny around unhealthy eating, they may resort to secretive eating habits. This behavior fosters a problematic relationship with food, marked by guilt and shame, further complicating the addiction cycle.

## Lifelong Consequences

- **Altered Taste Preferences**: Early and repeated exposure to the potent tastes of processed foods and sugars can dull the palate, making the subtle flavors of whole foods less appealing. This alteration can cement dietary preferences that favor unhealthy choices, perpetuating the cycle of addiction into adulthood.

- **Health Implications**: The chronic consumption of these foods lays the groundwork for a host of health issues, such as obesity, type 2 diabetes, and cardiovascular diseases. The management of these conditions often becomes a central aspect of life, reinforcing unhealthy coping mechanisms and perpetuating the cycle of addiction.

- **Social and Psychological Impact**: The stigma attached to poor dietary habits and resulting health conditions can lead to social isolation and diminished self-esteem. These emotional burdens can exacerbate food addiction, as individuals seek comfort and escape in the very foods contributing to their plight.

## Pathways to Intervention

- **Educational Initiatives**: Arming children and their families with knowledge about the nutritional content of foods and the importance of dietary choices is crucial. Programs that emphasize the value of whole foods and the dangers of excessive sugar and processed food consumption can lay the foundation for healthier lifelong eating habits.

- **Promotion of Healthy Coping Strategies**: Encouraging activities that provide emotional fulfillment beyond eating—such as sports, arts, and social engagement—can help children develop more constructive coping mechanisms.

- **Supportive Environments**: Creating environments that favor healthy eating choices, both at home and in schools, can significantly impact children's dietary habits. Limiting the availability of processed foods and ensuring access to nutritious options can help mitigate the allure of unhealthy foods.

It's imperative to recognize that the burgeoning addiction to processed foods and refined sugars among children is more than a mere health anomaly; it's a pressing psychological and societal issue. This chapter has delved into the multifaceted nature of this addiction, uncovering how it intertwines with physiological dependence, emotional reliance, cognitive conditioning, and ultimately manifests in behavioral shifts that can set the stage for a lifetime of unhealthy eating patterns. The comparison to substance addiction underscores the severity of this crisis, as children become ensnared in a cycle of cravings, emotional eating, and dietary habits that are hard to break.

Understanding the depth and breadth of food addiction in children sheds light on the urgent need for holistic intervention strategies. These must go beyond simple dietary guidelines, addressing the emotional, cognitive, and environmental factors that contribute to the development and perpetuation of these addictive behaviors. Educational initiatives that provide comprehensive knowledge about the impact of diet on health and well-being, alongside supportive environments that encourage healthy eating habits, are crucial steps forward. Moreover, promoting healthy coping mechanisms for emotional regulation without relying on food is essential for breaking the cycle of addiction.

As we move forward, it's clear that tackling processed food and sugar addiction in childhood requires a concerted effort from families, educators, policymakers, and the community at large. By fostering an environment that prioritizes nutritious, whole foods and supports children in developing a healthy relationship with food, we can begin to dismantle the maze of addiction. The goal is to empower children to make informed dietary choices, ensuring their path towards a healthy, fulfilling life is as clear and unobstructed as possible. Let this chapter serve as a call to action—to recognize the gravity of food addiction in childhood and to commit to the necessary steps to address it head-on, paving the way for healthier future generations.

# CHAPTER 6

## Unmasking the Shadow: *Chemicals and Dyes in Processed Foods— Implications for Child Development*

---

I n the era of convenience and fast food, processed foods have become an integral part of daily consumption, particularly among children. Yet, lurking beneath the surface of these seemingly benign products is a complex array of chemical additives and artificial dyes. These substances, while enhancing flavor, color, and shelf life, harbor potential risks that could significantly impact the developmental trajectory and overall health of children. This chapter delves into a shadowy side of processed foods, unraveling the intricate web of chemical culprits and their profound implications on the young, developing organism.

## The Array of Chemical Culprits

The modern processed food industry relies heavily on a spectrum of chemical additives to achieve the desired consumer appeal and product longevity. Among these are:

- **Artificial Dyes**: Colors like Red 40, Yellow 5, and Blue 1 are ubiquitous in children's foods, from candies to cereals. Despite their role in making products attractive, studies, such as those reviewed by the Center for Science in the Public Interest, have raised concerns about their links to behavioral issues, including hyperactivity and attention deficits in susceptible populations. Several studies have raised concerns about the potential cancer-causing effects of Red 40 dye. Animal studies have indicated that high doses of Red 40 can lead to the development of tumors. For example, some research has shown that consuming large amounts of food dyes, including Red 40, can promote tumor growth in rodents (Cleveland Clinic) (Pederson's Natural Farms) . Additionally, a study published on the impacts of Red 40 on human colon cancer cells revealed that the dye could cause DNA damage and colonic inflammation in mice, further supporting potential cancer risks (Pederson's Natural Farms) (CSPI).

- **Preservatives:** Sodium benzoate and butylated hydroxytoluene (BHT) are common preservatives with the potential to exacerbate asthma and cause other sensitivities. Research has indicated possible associations with cancer risk, urging a reevaluation of their safety in food.

These additives, while approved for use, have sparked a debate regarding their long-term effects on child health, with some studies suggesting detrimental impacts on behavior, cognitive function, and physical health.

# Foods and Beverages Containing Artificial Dyes

- **Candies and Sweets**: Many brightly colored candies are likely to contain artificial dyes like Red 40, Yellow 5, and Blue 1 to make them more appealing to children.

- **Soft Drinks and Fruit-flavored Beverages**: Some soft drinks and fruit-flavored beverages use artificial dyes to enhance their color, making them visually more attractive.

- **Cereals**: Certain breakfast cereals, especially those marketed towards children, often contain artificial colors to make them appear more fun and enticing.

- **Snack Foods**: Snack foods, including some chips and popcorn, may be colored with artificial dyes to improve their appearance.

- **Baked Goods**: Cookies, cakes, and pastries that are brightly colored are likely to contain one or more artificial dyes.

# Foods and Beverages Containing Preservatives

- **Soft Drinks**: Sodium benzoate is commonly found in acidic drinks like sodas to inhibit the growth of mold, yeast, and bacteria.

- **Packaged Snacks**: Butylated hydroxytoluene (BHT) is used in certain snack foods to prevent rancidity and extend shelf life. It can be found in items like chips and preserved pastries.

- **Condiments and Salad Dressings**: Sodium benzoate is also used in various condiments and salad dressings to enhance preservation.

- **Canned Foods**: Both sodium benzoate and BHT can be found in some canned foods to maintain freshness and prevent microbial growth.

While these additives have been approved for use by food safety authorities in many countries, ongoing research and public concern about their long-term health effects, especially on children, continue to fuel the debate over their safety.

Ten insights derived from various studies and reviews regarding the potential negative effects of artificial dyes on children:

1. **Behavioral Issues:** A notable study published in The *Lancet* in 2007 found that some children, especially those with existing behavioral disorders like ADHD, exhibited increased hyperactivity when consuming foods containing artificial dyes.

2. **Allergic Reactions:** Although relatively rare, some children may experience allergic reactions to certain artificial food dyes, including symptoms like hives, itchiness, and asthma. The prevalence of such allergic reactions is not well-defined but is a concern for susceptible individuals.

3. **Cancer Risk:** Research, including animal studies, has raised concerns about certain artificial dyes possibly being carcinogenic. For example, Red 3 (Erythrosine) has been linked to thyroid tumors in rats, as noted by the U.S. Food and

Drug Administration (FDA), prompting ongoing scrutiny and calls for further research into its safety.

4. **Increased Attention Deficit:** A meta-analysis conducted by researchers and published in the *Journal of the American Academy of Child & Adolescent Psychiatry* in 2012 reinforced the association between artificial food coloring and increased attention deficit in some children.

5. **Learning Impairment:** Some studies suggest a potential link between the consumption of artificial dyes and impaired learning ability, although this relationship requires further investigation to fully understand the impact and mechanisms involved.

6. **Environmental Impact:** Indirectly affecting children, the production and use of artificial dyes have environmental consequences, contributing to pollution and ecological disruption, which in turn can affect children's health and well-being.

7. **Dietary Quality:** Foods containing artificial dyes are often of lower nutritional value, contributing to poor dietary patterns among children. A diet high in such foods can lead to nutritional deficiencies and poor health outcomes over time.

8. **Gastrointestinal Distress:** Some anecdotal reports and preliminary studies have suggested that artificial dyes may cause or exacerbate gastrointestinal distress in some children, including symptoms like bloating and abdominal pain.

9. **Sleep Disturbances:** There is emerging evidence to suggest that artificial food dyes may impact children's

sleep patterns, potentially leading to difficulties in falling asleep or sleep disturbances, although this area is still under exploration.

10. **Potential for Long-term Health Effects:** The long-term health effects of artificial dyes on children are not fully understood, with concerns that continued exposure from a young age could contribute to chronic health issues later in life.

# Developmental and Growth Implications

## Cognitive and Neurological Development: The Crucial Role of Nutrition

The intricate process of brain development in children is a marvel of nature, finely tuned and remarkably sensitive to a host of environmental factors, including nutrition. Nutrients play a pivotal role in every stage of neurological development, from the formation of neural pathways to the myelination of neurons, which facilitates the rapid transmission of signals across the brain. This delicate developmental phase lays the foundation for cognitive abilities, learning, memory, and emotional regulation. However, the invasion of chemical additives and the overabundance of sugars in the modern diet threaten to disrupt this critical growth process, potentially leading to lasting cognitive deficits and neurological disturbances.

The prevalence of artificial dyes and preservatives in processed foods has become a significant concern for child health and development. These chemical additives, while enhancing the aesthetic appeal and shelf life of food products, may carry hidden costs for the developing brain. For instance, studies have linked certain artificial dyes to behavioral issues in children, including increased hyper-activity and reduced attention span. These effects are particularly concerning in the context of learning environments, where sustained attention and behavioral regulation are essential for academic success.

Preservatives, another common group of additives, have also come under scrutiny for their potential neurotoxic effects. Compounds such as sodium benzoate, commonly found in soft drinks and packaged snacks, have been associated with oxidative stress within neural cells, a condition that can lead to neuronal damage over time. This oxidative stress is thought to exacerbate neurodevelopmental disorders and may impair cognitive functions, highlighting the need for cautious consumption of foods containing these preservatives.

## The Sugar Dilemma

The high sugar content characteristic of many processed foods represents another threat to cognitive and neurological development. Sugars, particularly in the form of high-fructose corn syrup, are omnipresent in children's diets, from breakfast cereals to snack bars and beverages. The immediate effect of sugar consumption on children often manifests as a quick surge in energy, followed by a rapid decline, colloquially known as the "sugar crash." This cycle of hyperactivity followed by lethargy can disrupt a child's ability to maintain focus and engage in learning activities, impacting academic performance.

Beyond the immediate behavioral impacts, the long-term consumption of high-sugar diets has been implicated in more profound cognitive effects. Research suggests that excessive sugar intake can alter the structure and function of the brain, affecting areas critical for memory and executive function. For example, studies in both human and animal models have observed changes in the hippocampus, the brain region involved in learning and memory, following high sugar consumption. These changes can impede the ability to learn and retain information, posing significant challenges to educational achievement and cognitive development.

## Nurturing Cognitive Health through Nutrition

Addressing the challenges posed by chemical additives and high sugar content in children's diets necessitates a collective shift towards nutritional awareness and healthier eating practices. Prioritizing whole, nutrient-rich foods can provide the essential building blocks for brain development, supporting cognitive functions and promoting overall neurological health. Additionally, reducing the reliance on processed foods laden with artificial additives and sugars can help mitigate the risks to cognitive development, setting the stage for a healthier, more cognitively resilient generation.

## Endocrine Disruption and Physical Growth

Certain food additives possess endocrine-disrupting capabilities, interfering with hormone function and normal physical development. These disruptions can manifest in delayed or abnormal puberty, growth issues, and potentially long-term metabolic disorders, as outlined in studies examining the effects of phthalates and other chemicals found in processed foods.

The dialogue around the safety and impact of artificial dyes, preservatives, and high sugar content is not merely academic but underscores a pressing public health concern. The potential for these additives to negatively influence behavior, learning capabilities, and even the fundamental processes of cognitive and neurological development cannot be overstated. Moreover, the emerging evidence linking these chemicals to endocrine disruption and altered physical growth points to the need for a reevaluation of their presence in foods targeted toward children.

Navigating the future of food safety and child health necessitates a multi-faceted approach. It calls for increased scrutiny and regulation of chemical additives in the food supply, greater public awareness and education on the impacts of these substances, and a collective push towards dietary practices that prioritize whole, nutrient-dense foods. By fostering an environment that reduces children's exposure to potentially harmful chemicals and sugars, we can better support their developmental needs and promote a trajectory toward lifelong health and well-being.

# CHAPTER 7

## From Junk to Joy: *Embracing Healthier Alternatives to Processed Foods and Sugars for Families*

---

In the complex landscape of childhood nutrition, the search for wholesome alternatives to processed foods and hidden sugars stands as a testament to our commitment to nurturing not only the physical well-being but also the inherent joy of children. This chapter is a culinary journey, offering practical ways to keep our children nourished and joyful without relying on unhealthy options.

### 1. Embrace Whole Foods:

The foundation of a healthy diet is built on whole, unprocessed ingredients. Swap out processed snacks for vibrant fruits and vegetables. Instead of reaching for a bag of chips, consider apple slices with almond butter for a satisfying crunch and natural sweetness. Replace white rice with quinoa or brown rice, offering a whole grain alternative that's both nutritious and filling. For proteins, opt for grilled chicken breast or fish over processed deli meats, pairing them with a rainbow of vegetables for a colorful and wholesome meal.

## 2. Rediscover Homemade Delights:

Homemade cooking brings not only nutritional benefits but also the joy of creating something from scratch. Replace store-bought granola bars with homemade versions using oats, nuts, seeds, and natural sweeteners like honey or maple syrup. Bake cookies with whole wheat or almond flour and sweeten them with mashed bananas or applesauce instead of refined sugar. These homemade delights offer a healthier alternative to processed snacks, imbuing your kitchen with the warmth of home-cooked love.

## 3. Opt for Smart Swaps:

Intelligent substitutions can transform meals from nutritionally void to vibrant. Trade sugary sodas for sparkling water jazzed up with slices of cucumber, lemon, or frozen berries. Instead of a bag of processed snacks, try carrot or celery sticks with a side of hummus or a small portion of nuts. For breakfast, swap sugary cereals for oatmeal topped with fresh berries, a sprinkle of cinnamon, and a touch of honey for natural sweetness. These swaps not only enhance nutritional value but also introduce a variety of flavors to your child's palate.

## 4. Harness the Power of Natural Sweeteners:

In the quest to reduce refined sugars, natural sweeteners are invaluable. Maple syrup or honey can sweeten homemade baked goods, while dates blended into smoothies or dessert recipes add natural sweetness and texture. Bananas, with their natural sugars, can sweeten pancakes or muffins, offering a healthful twist on breakfast favorites. These natural sweeteners bring a depth of flavor and nutritional benefits, making them a superior choice for sweetening dishes.

## 5. Cultivate Culinary Curiosity:

Encouraging a spirit of culinary exploration can be a powerful tool in combating processed food consumption. Involve your children in meal planning and preparation, letting them discover the joy of cooking with whole foods. Experiment with making your own pizza with a whole wheat crust and fresh vegetable toppings instead of ordering out. Explore international cuisines that emphasize fresh ingredients and vibrant flavors, such as making a simple stir-fry with a variety of vegetables and a homemade sauce. This not only broadens their taste horizons but also instills a love for nutritious, homemade meals.

**Try the substitutions below.**

- Instead of sugary cereals try whole grain oats or homemade granola with nuts, seeds, and a bit of honey or maple syrup.

- Processed Chips ➡ Baked veggie chips (kale, sweet potato) or whole grain crackers with hummus or guacamole.

- Sugary Sodas ➡ Sparkling water with a splash of 100 percent fruit juice or infused with fresh fruit slices.

- Processed Snack Bars ➡ Homemade bars with oats, nuts, seeds, and dried fruits, bound together with honey or peanut butter.

- White Bread ➡ Whole grain or sprouted bread offering more fiber and nutrients.

- Store-Bought Cookies ➡ Homemade cookies made with whole grain flour, oats, and natural sweeteners like applesauce or ripe bananas.

- Ice Cream ➡ Blended frozen bananas for a creamy treat, or yogurt with fruit and a drizzle of honey.

- Candy ➡ Dried fruit like dates or figs for a natural sweet fix, or dark chocolate (70 percent or higher) for a healthier indulgence.

- Pre-Packaged Meals ➡ Home-cooked meals using whole ingredients, with spices and herbs for flavor instead of processed sauces.

- Sweetened Yogurt ➡ Plain Greek yogurt sweetened with fresh fruit or a touch of honey.

- Fruit Snacks ➡ Actual fresh fruit, or homemade fruit leather made by pureeing and baking fruit.

- Fried Chicken ➡ Oven-baked or air-fried chicken with a crunchy whole grain breadcrumb coating.

- Boxed Mac and Cheese ➡ Whole grain pasta with homemade cheese sauce using real cheese and milk.

These swaps not only reduce intake of processed foods and sugars but also enrich the diet with essential nutrients, promoting overall health and well-being.

## Crafting a Healthier Path: Junk Food Alternatives for Kids

In an era where convenience often dictates our dietary choices, it's increasingly challenging to navigate the labyrinth of food options, especially for our children. The allure of fast food, with its vibrant colors and instant gratification, is undeniable. Yet, as parents and caregivers, we face the daunting task of balancing convenience with nutrition, ensuring our children's health without depriving them of the joys of childhood treats. This chapter aims to guide you through the process of finding healthier alternatives to junk food, transforming temptation into an opportunity for nourishment and enjoyment.

## The Allure of Fast Food: A Double-Edged Sword

Fast food, a staple of modern diets, is often criticized for its high levels of sugar, unhealthy fats, and calories, all offering little in the way of essential nutrients. The temptation of these quick, tasty options is particularly strong among children, whose developing palates are easily swayed by the promise of immediate satisfaction. Recognizing this, the goal is not to eliminate these foods entirely but to moderate their consumption and make healthier choices whenever possible.

## Kid-Friendly Junk Food Alternatives

A crucial step in this journey is to identify alternatives that cater to children's preferences while prioritizing their health. Let's explore some simple swaps for popular junk food items:

- French Fries to Oven-Baked Fries: Transform the quintessential fast-food staple into a healthier version by baking thinly sliced potatoes in the oven. A light sprinkle of salt can enhance their natural flavors without overwhelming them.

- Ice Cream to Yogurt or Smoothies: Satisfy sweet cravings with yogurt or fresh fruit smoothies. These alternatives provide the creamy texture and sweetness children love, with the added benefits of probiotics and essential vitamins.

- Fried Chicken to Baked or Grilled Variants: By choosing to bake or grill chicken, you significantly reduce the fat content without sacrificing flavor, offering a protein-rich meal that's both delicious and nutritious.

- Doughnuts and Pastries to Home-Baked Goods: When the craving for something sweet and doughy strikes, opt for home-baked goods. By controlling the ingredients, you can reduce sugar levels and incorporate whole grains, creating a more balanced treat.

- Potato Chips to Baked Vegetable Chips or Nuts: For a crunchy snack, try baking thinly sliced vegetables or offering nuts to older children. These alternatives provide essential nutrients and healthy fats, making them a superior choice for snacking.

## Dining Out with Kids: Navigating the Menu

Eating out presents its own set of challenges, but with a bit of foresight, you can ensure a healthier dining experience:

- **Choose Healthier Sides:** Opt for grilled vegetables, side salads, or apple slices instead of calorie-laden options like fries or onion rings.

- **Watch Portion Sizes:** Stick to children's menus or smaller sizes to prevent overeating. Ordering pizza by the slice can satisfy cravings without leading to indulgence.

- **Opt for Nutritious Main Courses:** When available, choose dishes like chicken and vegetables over heavy, cheesy options like macaroni and cheese.

- **Make Smart Substitutions:** Don't hesitate to ask for healthier substitutes, especially in kid's meals. Replacing soda with water, and fries with fruits can make a significant difference.

We stand at the precipice of a transformative opportunity. This chapter serves not just as a guide but as an invitation to reimagine our approach to feeding our children, to replace convenience with conscious choice, and to elevate nutrition from a mere necessity to a source of joy and communal well-being. Through the exploration of whole foods, the rediscovery of homemade delights, smart swaps, the utilization of natural sweeteners, and the cultivation of culinary curiosity, we embark on a journey towards reclaiming the essence of nourishment.

This narrative encourages us not to view the shift away from processed foods and sugars as a loss but as a gain—an opportunity to instill lifelong habits of healthy eating, to awaken a sense of wonder in our children as they discover the true flavors of nature's bounty, and to forge deeper connections within our families through the shared experience of cooking and eating together. It emphasizes that the journey from junk to joy is paved with education, awareness, and creativity, inviting us to embrace the challenge as an act of love—a commitment to the future health and happiness of our children.

# CHAPTER 8

## Wholesome and Delicious Recipes for Children's Meals

---

In this chapter, we'll explore a selection of nutritious and kid-friendly recipes made with organic ingredients and limited added sugars. These recipes are designed to be budget-friendly and appeal to children's taste buds while providing essential nutrients for growth, development, and overall well-being. From breakfast to dinner and snacks in between, these recipes offer a variety of options to keep your child's diet balanced and delicious.

## 1. *Breakfast*: Banana Oatmeal Pancakes

Ingredients

- 1 ripe banana, mashed
- 1 cup rolled oats
- 1/2 cup milk (dairy or plant-based)
- 1 egg
- 1 teaspoon vanilla extract

- 1/2 teaspoon cinnamon

- 1/4 teaspoon baking powder

- Pinch of salt

## Instructions

1. In a blender or food processor, combine all ingredients and blend until smooth.

2. Heat a non-stick skillet over medium heat and lightly coat with cooking spray or butter.

3. Pour batter onto the skillet to form small pancakes.

4. Cook until bubbles form on the surface, then flip and cook until golden brown on both sides.

5. Serve with fresh fruit and a drizzle of pure maple syrup or yogurt.

# 2. *Lunch*: Veggie and Hummus Wrap

## Ingredients

- Whole grain tortilla wraps

- Hummus

- Sliced cucumbers

- Shredded carrots

- Sliced bell peppers

- Baby spinach or mixed greens

Instructions

1. Spread a generous layer of hummus onto a tortilla wrap.

2. Layer sliced vegetables on top of the hummus.

3. Add a handful of baby spinach or mixed greens.

4. Roll up the wrap tightly and slice into bite-sized pieces.

5. Serve with a side of sliced fruit or vegetable sticks and a dip like yogurt or guacamole.

## 3. *Snack*: Ants on a Log

Ingredients:

- Celery stalks
- Peanut butter or almond butter
- Raisins

Instructions:

1. Cut celery stalks into manageable lengths.

2. Spread peanut butter or almond butter onto each celery stalk.

3. Place raisins on top of the nut butter to resemble "ants" on a log.

4. Serve as a fun and nutritious snack that kids can assemble themselves.

## 4. *Dinner*: Turkey and Veggie Meatballs with Whole Wheat Pasta

Ingredients**:**

- 1 pound lean ground turkey
- 1/2 cup finely grated zucchini
- 1/2 cup finely grated carrots
- 1/4 cup whole wheat breadcrumbs
- 1 egg
- 2 cloves garlic, minced
- 1 teaspoon Italian seasoning
- Salt and pepper to taste
- Whole wheat pasta, cooked according to package instructions
- Marinara sauce (store-bought or homemade)

Instructions**:**

1. Preheat oven to 375°F (190°C) and line a baking sheet with parchment paper.

2. In a large bowl, combine ground turkey, grated zucchini, grated carrots, breadcrumbs, egg, minced garlic, Italian seasoning, salt, and pepper. Mix until well combined.

3. Roll mixture into meatballs and place them on the prepared baking sheet.

4. Bake for 20 to 25 minutes, or until meatballs are cooked through and lightly browned.

5. Serve meatballs over cooked whole wheat pasta with marinara sauce. Optionally, sprinkle with grated Parmesan cheese.

## 5. *Dessert*: Fruit Salad with Honey Lime Dressing

Ingredients:

- Assorted fresh fruits (such as strawberries, blueberries, grapes, pineapple, and kiwi), chopped
- 2 tablespoons honey
- Juice of 1 lime
- Fresh mint leaves, chopped (optional)

Instructions:

1. In a large bowl, combine chopped fruits.
2. In a small bowl, whisk together honey and lime juice to make the dressing.
3. Pour the dressing over the fruit and gently toss to coat.
4. Garnish with chopped mint leaves, if desired.
5. Serve immediately or refrigerate until ready to enjoy.

## 1. *Breakfast*: Berry Banana Smoothie Bowl

Ingredients:

- 1 ripe banana, frozen
- 1 cup mixed berries (such as strawberries, blueberries, and raspberries), frozen

- 1/2 cup plain Greek yogurt

- 1/4 cup milk (dairy or plant-based)

- 1 tablespoon honey or maple syrup (optional)

- Toppings: granola, sliced fruit, shredded coconut, chia seeds

Instructions:

1. In a blender, combine frozen banana, frozen berries, Greek yogurt, and milk. Blend until smooth and creamy.

2. If desired, sweeten with honey or maple syrup to taste.

3. Pour the smoothie into a bowl and top with granola, sliced fruit, shredded coconut, and chia seeds for added texture and flavor.

4. Serve immediately and enjoy with a spoon.

## 2. *Lunch*: Quinoa Salad with Chickpeas and Veggies

Ingredients:

- 1 cup cooked quinoa, cooled

- 1 can chickpeas, drained and rinsed

- 1 cup cherry tomatoes, halved

- 1 cucumber, diced

- 1/4 cup red onion, finely chopped

- 1/4 cup fresh parsley, chopped

- 2 tablespoons olive oil

- 1 tablespoon lemon juice
- Salt and pepper to taste

Instructions:

1. In a large bowl, combine cooked quinoa, chickpeas, cherry tomatoes, cucumber, red onion, and parsley.

2. In a small bowl, whisk together olive oil, lemon juice, salt, and pepper to make the dressing.

3. Pour the dressing over the quinoa salad and toss until well coated.

4. Serve as a nutritious and satisfying lunch option.

# 3. *Snack*: Apple Sandwiches with Peanut Butter and Granola

Ingredients:

- 1 apple, cored and sliced horizontally into rounds
- Peanut butter or almond butter
- Granola
- Optional additions: raisins, shredded coconut, chocolate chips

Instructions:

1. Spread peanut butter or almond butter onto one side of each apple slice.

2. Sprinkle granola over the nut butter, pressing lightly to adhere.

3. If desired, add additional toppings such as raisins, shredded coconut, or chocolate chips.

4. Sandwich two apple slices together to form "apple sandwiches."

5. Serve as a fun and nutritious snack that's perfect for on-the-go.

# 4. *Dinner*: Veggie-Packed Turkey Chili

Ingredients:

- 1 tablespoon olive oil
- 1 onion, diced
- 2 cloves garlic, minced
- 1 pound lean ground turkey
- 1 bell pepper, diced
- 1 zucchini, diced
- 1 carrot, diced
- 1 can (15 ounces) diced tomatoes
- 1 can (15 ounces) black beans, drained and rinsed
- 1 cup low-sodium chicken broth
- 2 tablespoons chili powder
- 1 teaspoon cumin
- Salt and pepper to taste
- Optional toppings: shredded cheese, avocado, Greek yogurt, cilantro

Instructions**:**

1. In a large pot, heat olive oil over medium heat. Add diced onion and garlic, and sauté until softened.

2. Add ground turkey to the pot and cook until browned, breaking it up with a spoon.

3. Stir in diced bell pepper, zucchini, and carrot, and cook for a few minutes until vegetables begin to soften.

4. Add diced tomatoes, black beans, chicken broth, chili powder, cumin, salt, and pepper to the pot. Stir to combine.

5. Bring the chili to a simmer and let it cook for 20 to 30 minutes, until flavors have melded and vegetables are tender.

6. Serve hot, garnished with shredded cheese, avocado slices, Greek yogurt, and fresh cilantro if desired.

# 5. *Dessert*: Yogurt Parfait with Berries and Granola

Ingredients**:**

- Greek yogurt (plain or flavored)

- Mixed berries (such as strawberries, blueberries, and raspberries)

- Granola

- Optional additions: honey, shredded coconut, chopped nuts

Instructions**:**

1. In a serving glass or bowl, layer Greek yogurt, mixed berries, and granola.

2. Repeat the layers until the glass is filled, ending with a layer of granola on top.

3. Drizzle with honey if desired and sprinkle with shredded coconut or chopped nuts for added crunch.

4. Serve immediately as a nutritious and satisfying dessert option.

# 1. *Breakfast*: Sweet Potato and Apple Muffins

Ingredients**:**

- 1 cup whole wheat flour

- 1/2 cup oat flour

- 1 teaspoon baking powder

- 1/2 teaspoon baking soda

- 1 teaspoon cinnamon

- 1/4 teaspoon nutmeg

- 1/2 cup unsweetened applesauce

- 1 cup sweet potato, cooked and mashed

- 1/4 cup maple syrup

- 2 eggs

- 1/4 cup milk (dairy or plant-based)

- 1/2 cup diced apples

Instructions:

1. Preheat the oven to 350°F (175°C) and line a muffin tin with paper liners.

2. In a large bowl, whisk together the whole wheat flour, oat flour, baking powder, baking soda, cinnamon, and nutmeg.

3. In another bowl, mix the applesauce, mashed sweet potato, maple syrup, eggs, and milk until well combined.

4. Fold the wet ingredients into the dry ingredients until just mixed. Gently stir in the diced apples.

5. Spoon the batter into the muffin tin and bake for 20 to 25 minutes, or until a toothpick inserted into the center comes out clean.

6. Allow to cool before serving. These muffins are a great way to start the day with fiber, vitamins, and a touch of sweetness.

## 2. *Lunch*: Chicken and Avocado Roll-Ups

Ingredients:

- Whole grain tortillas
- 1 cup cooked and shredded chicken
- 1 ripe avocado, mashed
- 1/4 cup shredded carrots
- 1/4 cup shredded cheese (optional)
- Baby spinach leaves

Instructions:

1. Spread a layer of mashed avocado onto a tortilla.

2. Add shredded chicken, carrots, cheese (if using), and a few spinach leaves on top of the avocado.

3. Roll up the tortilla tightly, then slice into bite-sized roll-ups.

4. Serve with a side of mixed fruit for a balanced and appealing lunch option.

# 3. *Snack*: Baked Sweet Potato Fries

Ingredients:

- 2 large sweet potatoes, peeled and cut into sticks
- 1 tablespoon olive oil
- 1 teaspoon paprika
- Salt to taste

Instructions:

1. Preheat the oven to 400°F (200°C) and line a baking sheet with parchment paper.

2. Toss sweet potato sticks with olive oil, paprika, and salt until evenly coated.

3. Spread the sweet potato sticks in a single layer on the baking sheet.

4. Bake for 25 to 30 minutes, turning once, until crispy and golden.

5. Cool slightly before serving. These fries offer a healthier alternative to traditional fried snacks, packed with vitamins and fiber.

## 4. *Dinner*: Cheesy Broccoli and Rice Casserole

Ingredients:

- 1 cup brown rice, cooked
- 2 cups broccoli florets, steamed
- 1 cup shredded cheese (Cheddar or mozzarella works well)
- 1/2 cup Greek yogurt
- 1/4 cup milk (dairy or plant-based)
- Salt and pepper to taste
- 1/4 teaspoon garlic powder

Instructions:

1. Preheat the oven to 375°F (190°C).

2. In a large bowl, mix the cooked rice, steamed broccoli, half of the cheese, Greek yogurt, milk, salt, pepper, and garlic powder.

3. Transfer the mixture to a greased baking dish and sprinkle the remaining cheese on top.

4. Bake for 20 to 25 minutes, or until the cheese is bubbly and golden.

5. Serve warm. This comforting casserole is a delicious way to get kids to enjoy their greens, with the creamy, cheesy rice ensuring they ask for seconds.

## 5. *Dessert*: Frozen Banana Yogurt Bites

Ingredients:

- 2 bananas, sliced
- 1/2 cup Greek yogurt

These recipes provide nutritious and delicious options for children's meals while emphasizing the use of organic ingredients and limited added sugars. By incorporating these wholesome recipes into your child's diet, you can promote healthy eating habits and support their overall well-being from an early age.

## Nurturing Growth: Wholesome Foods and Supplements for Kids on a Budget

Raising a healthy family in today's fast-paced world, where processed foods and high sugar content dominate, can be a formidable challenge, especially for parents with multiple kids and tight budgets. This chapter offers a comprehensive guide to navigating this landscape, focusing on budget-friendly, nutritious food and supplement choices that cater to the needs of growing children without compromising on quality or health.

## Embracing the Essentials:
## Fruits, Vegetables, and Whole Grains

The foundation of a healthy diet for children revolves around fruits, vegetables, and whole grains. These food groups are not only packed with essential nutrients for growth and development but are also remarkably wallet-friendly, especially when seasonal produce is chosen or purchased in bulk.

- **Seasonal Strategies:** Leveraging seasonal fruits and vegetables can significantly reduce costs. Community-supported agriculture (CSA) programs or local farmers' markets often offer fresh produce at lower prices than supermarkets. The following page can help locate CSA's in your area : www.LocalHarvest.org

- **Whole Grain Wisdom:** Foods like oats, brown rice, and whole wheat pasta are not only nutritious and filling but also cost-effective. Buying these in bulk can further stretch your dollar, providing a healthy base for meals that can be flavored and varied in countless ways.

## Protein and Dairy: Affordable Options

Protein is crucial for children's growth, but it doesn't have to come with a high price tag. Eggs, legumes, and canned fish offer high-quality protein at a fraction of the cost of fresh meat or fish. Similarly, dairy and its alternatives provide necessary calcium and vitamin D, with many budget-friendly options available.

- **Creative Cooking:** Eggs and legumes can be turned into various delicious, child-friendly dishes, from scrambled eggs to lentil patties. Likewise, dairy products like yogurt and cheese can be bought in larger, generic brand containers to save money without sacrificing nutritional value.

## Supplements: A Cost-Effective Safety Net

While a balanced diet is paramount, supplements can play a critical role in ensuring children get all the nutrients they need, particularly when dietary restrictions or health conditions are present. Choosing the right supplements involves a focus on quality, necessity, and budget.

- **Selective Supplementation:** Key supplements like multivitamins, vitamin D, omega-3 fatty acids, iron, and calcium can fill nutritional gaps. Opting for generic brands, buying in bulk, and prioritizing essential nutrients can make supplementation both effective and economical. We'll take an in-depth look at supplements in the following chapter.

- **Safety and Efficacy:** Always consult a healthcare provider before introducing supplements to ensure they are necessary and safe. Paying attention to recommended dosages and potential allergens is crucial to avoid adverse effects.

# Budget-Friendly Strategies for a Healthy Family

Feeding a family nutritiously on a budget requires creativity, planning, and a bit of savvy shopping. Here are some additional tips to maximize nutrition while minimizing costs:

- **Meal Planning:** Plan meals around seasonal produce and sales on whole grains and proteins. Preparing larger batches of meals that can be frozen or used throughout the week can save both time and money.

- **Educational Engagement:** Involving kids in meal planning and preparation can increase their interest in healthy eating. It's also an excellent opportunity to teach them about nutrition and budgeting.

- **Smart Shopping:** Keep an eye out for discounts, use coupons, and consider store or generic brands for both food and supplements. These often offer the same nutritional value at a lower cost.

As we end on chapter 8, we're reminded of the profound impact our culinary choices have on the health and happiness of our children. Through the selection of nutritious, kid-friendly recipes detailed in this chapter, we've embarked on a flavorful journey that prioritizes whole, organic ingredients and minimizes added sugars—proving that nourishment and delight can coexist on our children's plates. These recipes are not just meals; they're an investment in our children's growth, development, and well-being, offering a palette of flavors and nutrients essential for their thriving bodies and minds.

From the simplicity of Banana Oatmeal Pancakes to the heartiness of Turkey and Veggie Meatballs with Whole Wheat Pasta, each recipe is a testament to the joy that wholesome food can bring into our lives. By embracing the principles of homemade cooking, smart swaps, and natural sweeteners, we can transform everyday meals from mere sustenance to moments of joy and exploration. This chapter encourages us to step beyond the convenience of processed options and discover the satisfaction of crafting meals that are both nutritious and delicious, fostering a love for healthy eating in our children that will last a lifetime.

Let this chapter serve as a beacon for families navigating the challenges of modern diets, offering practical solutions and inspiring ideas to make healthy eating accessible, enjoyable, and, above all, delicious. By choosing to embrace these recipes and the principles they embody, we commit to a future where our children are not only well-fed but also well-nourished, equipped with the tastes and habits that will support their health and happiness for years to come.

# CHAPTER 9

## Essential Supplements and Nutrient-Rich Foods for Children

---

I n the journey towards nurturing a healthy and vibrant child, the role of proper nutrition cannot be overstated. While a balanced diet is paramount, certain supplements can fill in nutritional gaps, ensuring that children receive all the nutrients they need for optimal growth and development. Below, we explore essential supplements for children, foods that naturally support these supplements for those who may struggle with pills, and a selection of healthy protein shakes and powders tailored for the younger palate.

## Essential Supplements for Daily Intake

**1. Vitamin D:** Essential for bone health and immune function, Vitamin D can be challenging to obtain through diet alone. Supplementing with Vitamin D ensures proper bone development and support.

- **Foods Rich in Vitamin D:** Fortified plant-based milks, mushrooms exposed to sunlight, and fatty fish like salmon and mackerel.

REF: https://pubmed.ncbi.nlm.nih.gov/20229973/
https://pubmed.ncbi.nlm.nih.gov/34815552/

**2. Omega-3 Fatty Acids (DHA and EPA):** Crucial for brain and eye development, Omega-3s are often lacking in children's diets. A supplement can support cognitive development and heart health.

- **Foods Rich in Omega-3s:** Chia seeds, flaxseeds, hemp seeds, walnuts, avocado, and fatty fish.

REF: https://pubmed.ncbi.nlm.nih.gov/28741625/
https://pubmed.ncbi.nlm.nih.gov/30594823/

**3. Iron:** Important for energy levels and cognitive development, iron is a critical supplement for children, especially those not consuming enough from their diet.

- **Foods Rich in Iron:** Lentils, beans, spinach, and iron-fortified cereals.

**4. Vitamin C:** This antioxidant supports the immune system and helps with the absorption of iron from plant-based sources.

- **Foods Rich in Vitamin C:** Oranges, strawberries, bell peppers, and kiwi.

REF: https://pubmed.ncbi.nlm.nih.gov/36364865/

**5. Probiotics:** These beneficial bacteria are crucial for maintaining a healthy gut microbiome, which supports digestive health and bolsters the immune system. Probiotics can help reduce the occurrence of diarrhea, constipation, and infections in children by enhancing gut flora balance and function.

- **Foods Rich in Probiotics:** Yogurt, kefir, sauerkraut, and other fermented foods.

For Vitamin D and Omega-3 supplements suitable for children, including those focused on supporting bone health, immune function, brain, and eye development, here are some recommended products along with links to where they can be purchased. Please ensure you consult with a healthcare provider before starting any new supplement regimen for your child.

## Vitamin D Supplements for Kids:

1. Nordic Naturals Vitamin D3 Gummies Kids - These gummies provide 400 IU of vitamin D3 in a tasty, chewable form that kids love. They're non-GMO, gluten-free, and dairy-free.

2. Carlson Kid's Vitamin D3 Drops - These drops offer 400 IU of vitamin D3 per drop, making it easy to adjust dosages. The drops can be added to food or drinks.

## Omega-3 Fatty Acids Supplements for Kids:

1. Nordic Naturals Children's DHA - Made from Arctic cod liver oil, these soft gels or liquid provide DHA and EPA, essential for brain development. They come in a strawberry flavor to appeal to kids.

2. Coromega Kids Omega-3 Fish Oil Squeeze Packets - These packets contain a creamy, flavored fish oil that's fun for kids to take. They offer a high dose of DHA and EPA without the fishy taste.

## Iron Supplements for Kids:

1. Renzo's Iron Strong, Vegan Dissolvable Vitamins for Kids - These are gentle on the stomach and specifically formulated for kids, providing an optimal dose of iron in a melt-in-your-mouth tablet.

2. NovaFerrum Pediatric Liquid Iron Supplement- This liquid supplement is naturally sweetened and offers a high bio-availability form of iron without the use of artificial colors or flavors.

## Vitamin C Supplements for Kids:

1. L'il Critters Immune C Plus Zinc & Echinacea - This gummy supplement combines vitamin C with zinc and echinacea to support the immune system in a form that's tasty and easy for kids to take.

2. MaryRuth's Vitamin C Gummies for Kids - These organic, vegan gummies provide vitamin C from organic acerola cherries. They're designed to be easy on the stomach and free from common allergens.

## Probiotic supplements for kids:

When looking for a probiotic supplement for kids, it's essential to choose a product that is specifically formulated for children, ensuring it has the appropriate strains and dosages suitable for their age and digestive system. One highly regarded option is:

### Culturelle Kids Daily Probiotic Packets

- Key Features: Culturelle Kids Daily Probiotic Packets are designed to help support kids' natural defense systems and reduce occasional digestive upset. They contain Lactobacillus rhamnosus GG, a clinically proven strain that survives the stomach's harsh environment.

- Benefits: This probiotic supplement can help with the digestive health of children, supporting a healthy balance of gut bacteria which is crucial for a functioning immune system and overall health. It's particularly noted for its ability to reduce the duration and severity of diarrhea, as well as aid in the overall digestive comfort.

- Usage: The packets are convenient and easy to use, making them a good option for busy families. They can be mixed into cold foods or beverages, which is helpful for kids who might be picky eaters or reluctant to take pills.

- Safety: Culturelle is a well-known brand that places a high emphasis on the purity and potency of its products. The packets are free from gluten, dairy, and sugar, catering to children with dietary restrictions.

Remember, it's important to consult with a pediatrician or a healthcare provider to determine the right dosage and type of supplement that is best suited for your child's health needs and dietary restrictions.

## Foods as Supplement Alternatives

For children who cannot swallow pills, incorporating nutrient-rich foods is a practical and effective strategy. Smoothies are an excellent vehicle for combining several of these foods into a delicious and nutritious treat. For example, a smoothie made with spinach, flaxseeds, and fortified plant-based milk can provide a good mix of iron, Omega-3s, and Vitamin D.

## Healthy Protein Shakes and Powders for Kids

When selecting protein shakes and powders, it's crucial to opt for products with no processed foods or added sugars. Look for shakes that use natural ingredients and are specifically formulated for children. Some healthy options include:

1. **Pea Protein Powders:** A great plant-based protein source that's easy to digest and often hypoallergenic, making it suitable for most children.

2. **Brown Rice Protein:** Another excellent plant-based option that can be easily mixed into smoothies and baked goods.

**Homemade Protein Shake Recipe:** Blend together one ripe banana, a handful of spinach, a tablespoon of unsweetened peanut or almond butter, a scoop of pea or brown rice protein powder, and a cup of fortified plant-based milk. This shake is not only delicious but also packs a nutritional punch, providing protein, iron, Vitamin D, and Omega-3s.

I found several recommended protein shakes and powders suitable for kids, highlighting their benefits and flavor profiles, ensuring they are aligned with preferences for natural ingredients and no added sugars.

1. Safe and Fair Kids Protein Powder offers a vegan, gluten-free option with pea protein, fiber, prebiotics, and

probiotics, making it allergy-friendly and beneficial for digestive health. It has a plant-based flavor that some kids may need to get used to. https://proteinsnackfinder.com/best-protein-shakes-and-powders-for-kids/.

2. Horizon Organic Whole Milk and Fairlife DHA Omega-3 are dairy-based options that provide a good source of protein, calcium, and vitamins. They are especially suitable for children without dairy allergies or lactose intolerance. Fairlife's milk is ultra-filtered to offer more protein and includes DHA Omega-3 for additional brain health benefits. https://proteinsnackfinder.com/best-protein-shakes-and-powders-for-kids/

3. Transparent Labs Grass-Fed Whey is highly recommended for its purity, containing no artificial sweeteners, food dyes, gluten, or preservatives. It's made from naturally fed, hormone-free cow whey, offering a high protein content with minimal calories. It comes in flavors like chocolate, strawberry, french vanilla, and salted caramel, catering to various tastes. https://totalshape.com/supplements/best-protein-powder-for-kids/

4. Ladder Whey Protein is praised for its taste, even without artificial sweeteners, and includes probiotics. Created by renowned personalities, it aims to support cognitive function and linear growth, offering flavors like chocolate and vanilla. https://totalshape.com/supplements/best-protein-powder-for-kids/

5. Ora Organic So Lean & So Clean stands out as an organic, vegan-friendly option, focusing on plant-based ingredients without artificial additives. https://totalshape.com/supplements/best-protein-powder-for-kids/

6. Drink Wholesome Chocolate Protein Powder is made with real food ingredients like powdered and dried egg whites, catering to a child's digestive system. It offers versatility in use, being suitable for smoothies, oatmeal, and pancakes, with classic flavors such as chocolate and vanilla. https://parenthoodbliss.com/protein-shakes-for-kids/

7. Amazing Grass KIDZ Superfood combines protein with probiotics, using organic ingredients like banana, beet juice powder, pineapple, and cocoa. It's a lower-calorie option that avoids artificial colors, flavors, or fillers, available in chocolate and strawberry flavors. https://parenthoodbliss.com/protein-shakes-for-kids/

When considering protein supplements for your child, it's essential to prioritize products that match their dietary needs and preferences, focusing on those with natural ingredients and minimal additives. Always consult with a healthcare provider to ensure these supplements are appropriate for your child's health and nutritional requirements.

As chapter 9 concludes, we're reminded of the delicate balance and critical importance of ensuring our children receive the nutrients they need for optimal growth, development, and overall health. This chapter has shed light on the essential supplements that can help fill nutritional gaps in our children's diets, alongside highlighting foods rich in these vital nutrients for those who may prefer or need alternatives to supplements. Moreover, the introduction of healthy protein shakes and powders tailored for young tastes underscores the possibility of blending nutritional necessity with palatable pleasure, ensuring that our children's journey towards health doesn't have to forsake enjoyment. By embracing a holistic approach to nutrition that combines a balanced diet with targeted supplementation, when necessary, we can lay a strong foundation for our children's future well-being.

The recipes and recommendations provided here serve not just as a guide but as a testament to the power of informed and mindful nutritional choices. As parents and caregivers, our role in shaping our children's dietary habits is profound, offering an opportunity to instill a love for wholesome, nutritious foods that will support their growth and serve their health throughout their lives.

Let this chapter be a resource and inspiration for families seeking to navigate the nutritional landscape with confidence and joy. By prioritizing essential nutrients, whether through food, supplements, or a combination of both, we can ensure our children are not just well-fed but well-nourished, ready to explore the world with energy, vitality, and a robust foundation of health.

# CHAPTER 10

## Broadening Horizons: *Encouraging Picky Eaters to Embrace Variety*

---

Navigating the dining table with a picky eater can often feel like steering through a stormy sea—unpredictable, challenging, and at times, downright daunting. The journey of expanding a child's palate is akin to a delicate dance, requiring patience, creativity, and a dash of strategy. Understanding that pickiness is a natural part of childhood development is the first step towards embracing and, ultimately, diversifying the range of foods your child enjoys.

### Understanding Picky Eaters

Picky eating is a common phase for many children, often reflecting their growing independence and developing taste preferences. Like adults who may hesitate before trying new cuisines, children require time and repeated exposure to familiarize themselves with and accept new flavors and textures. Research suggests that it may take between eight to ten presentations of a new food before a child decides to accept it. Patience, therefore, becomes a key ingredient in the recipe for success.

## Strategies for Expanding the Palate

Rather than a one-size-fits-all approach, encouraging children to explore a variety of foods involves a blend of tactics tailored to their individual responses and preferences. Here are some strategies to help make mealtime less of a battleground and more of an adventure:

- **Capitalize on Hunger:** Offer new foods when your child is most hungry, and limit snacks throughout the day to ensure they have an appetite come mealtime.

- **Introduce One New Food at a Time:** Avoid overwhelming your child by presenting only one new food alongside familiar favorites. This can help them focus on the new experience without feeling pressured.

- **Engage Their Sense of Fun:** Children are more likely to try new foods when the experience feels playful. Use cookie cutters to shape fruits and vegetables into fun figures, or arrange the plate into a colorful landscape, making mealtime both imaginative and enticing.

- **Combine New with Known:** Serving new foods alongside well-loved favorites can help reduce apprehension. Incorporating vegetables into a favorite soup or mixing a new grain into a beloved stew can subtly introduce new tastes and textures.

- **Involve Them in Meal Preparation:** Children take pride in their creations. By involving them in the cooking process, from picking recipes to preparing dishes, they're more likely to be curious and excited about tasting the outcome.

- **Mind the Beverages and Snacks:** Limiting beverages and snacks between meals ensures that children come to the table with an appetite, making them more open to trying new foods.

Some other strategies to consider:

- **Leverage Hunger:** Use moments of heightened hunger to introduce new foods, ensuring snacks are moderated throughout the day to cultivate a hearty appetite at meal times.

- **Incremental Introductions:** To prevent overwhelming your child, introduce a single new item amidst familiar favorites, providing a focused yet low-pressure exposure to the new food.

- **Fostering Fun and Imagination:** Mealtime becomes an enticing adventure when infused with elements of play. Transform fruits and vegetables with cookie cutters into engaging shapes or assemble meals into vibrant, appealing scenes that captivate their imagination and curiosity.

- **Blending the New with the Familiar:** Introducing new foods alongside beloved ones can reduce apprehension. For instance, integrating a novel vegetable into a favored soup or a new grain into a cherished stew can subtly acquaint them with diverse tastes and textures.

- **Culinary Participation:** Involving children in meal planning and preparation, from selecting recipes to assisting in the kitchen, enhances their eagerness and openness to taste their creations.

- **Optimizing Beverages and Snacks:** Regulating liquid consumption and snacks between meals guarantees that children approach the dining table eager and ready to explore new flavors.

## The Power of Positive Modeling

Children learn by example, making the eating habits and attitudes of parents and caregivers incredibly influential. Demonstrating a willingness to try new foods yourself can inspire your child to do the same. Share your enthusiasm for the flavors and stories behind different dishes, making each new food an adventure rather than a chore.

## Embracing Patience and Persistence

It's important to remember that expanding a child's dietary repertoire is a gradual process, filled with successes and setbacks. Celebrate the small victories, such as when they're willing to try a bite of something new, and don't be disheartened by the inevitable rejections. With time, patience, and consistent effort, picky eaters can learn to enjoy a wider variety of foods, paving the way for a lifetime of healthy, adventurous eating.

As we wrap up Chapter 10, it's clear that the path to diversifying a child's palate is much more an art than a science, blending patience, creativity, and understanding into the daily rhythm of meals. This journey, while sometimes fraught with setbacks, offers an invaluable opportunity to instill in children a lifelong appreciation for the richness of diverse foods and the benefits of a balanced diet. By approaching picky eating not as a hurdle but as a natural phase of childhood development, we can employ strategies that gradually introduce new flavors and textures in a manner that respects each child's pace and preferences.

The strategies outlined in this chapter—from leveraging hunger to making mealtime playful and involving children in the culinary process—underscore the importance of a thoughtful, tailored approach to expanding a child's dietary horizons. Moreover, the power of positive modeling by parents and caregivers cannot be overstated, as children are keen observers, often mirroring the eating habits and attitudes toward food they see at home.

In addition to the useful information provided in this chapter, a great resource for addressing picky eating in children is the website Nutrition for Littles. This site focuses on practical solutions and strategies to help parents and caregivers manage and overcome picky eating habits. You can find more tips and guidance at Nutrition for Littles https://nutritionforlittles.com .

Ultimately, the goal is not merely to conquer picky eating but to foster a sense of curiosity and openness in children toward trying new foods, setting the foundation for a healthy relationship with eating that prioritizes nourishment and enjoyment in equal measure. By celebrating the small victories and maintaining a steady course through the occasional challenges, we can guide our children toward a world of culinary diversity that enriches both their bodies and their spirits. Let this chapter serve as a beacon for parents navigating the waters of picky eating, offering hope, inspiration, and practical advice for turning mealtime from a battleground into a journey of discovery and delight.

# CHAPTER 11

# Fun and Effective Workouts for Kids

---

In today's world, where technology often dominates children's leisure time, it's more important than ever to encourage physical activity. However, traditional workouts might not be appealing to kids. That's where creative and enjoyable workouts come into play. In this chapter, we'll explore a variety of workouts tailored specifically for children aged six to fifteen years old, utilizing bodyweight exercises and items found around the house or outdoors. These workouts are designed to be fun, engaging, and effective, promoting not only physical fitness but also a sense of enjoyment and accomplishment.

## 1. Warm-Up Activities:

Before diving into the workouts, it's crucial to start with a proper warm-up to prepare the body for exercise. Here are some fun warm-up activities for kids:

- Jumping jacks

- High knees

- Arm circles

- Toe touches

- Jogging in place

## 2. Circuit Training:

Circuit training involves moving through a series of exercises with little to no rest in between. Set up stations around your backyard or living room and have the kids rotate through them. Here's a sample circuit:

- Station 1: Jump rope (use a real jump rope or pretend with an imaginary one)

- Station 2: Hula hoop (see how long they can keep it spinning!)

- Station 3: Chair squats (use a sturdy chair)

- Station 4: Bear crawls (crawl on all fours like a bear)

- Station 5: Plank hold (see who can hold it the longest)

## 3. Obstacle Course:

Create an obstacle course using household items and outdoor space. Incorporate tasks like crawling under tables, jumping over pillows, and weaving through cones. Time each child as they navigate the course, encouraging friendly competition and improvement.

## 4. Yoga and Stretching:

Yoga is a fantastic way to improve flexibility, balance, and mindfulness. Choose kid-friendly yoga poses such as downward dog, tree pose, and cobra. Encourage deep breathing and relaxation as they flow through the poses. After yoga, lead them through some simple stretching exercises to cool down and prevent muscle soreness.

## 5. Outdoor Adventures:

Take advantage of outdoor spaces for active play. Here are some ideas:

- **Bike riding:** Explore the neighborhood on bikes or scooters.
- **Nature scavenger hunt:** Create a list of items for the kids to find, such as rocks, leaves, and flowers.
- **Playground fun:** Head to the local playground for climbing, swinging, and sliding.
- **Ball games:** Play soccer, basketball, or catch with a ball or frisbee.

## 6. Dance Party:

Crank up the music and have a dance party! Encourage the kids to let loose and move to the beat. Dance is a fantastic cardiovascular workout and a fun way to express creativity.

## 7. Chores with a Twist:

Turn household chores into a workout by adding some fun challenges. For example, see who can sweep the floor the fastest or do the most jumping jacks while folding laundry.

Here are ten additional ways to keep children active, focusing on variety and fun to spark their interest and maintain their engagement:

1. **Nature Hikes:** Exploring local trails or parks on foot is a great way for kids to connect with nature while getting their steps in. Make it educational by identifying different types of plants, birds, and insects.

2. **Water Play:** Swimming, water polo, or even simple games in a pool encourage vigorous physical activity while providing a cool respite on hot days. For those without pool access, running through sprinklers or having a water balloon toss are enjoyable alternatives.

3. **Team Sports:** Joining local soccer, baseball, or basketball leagues not only promotes physical activity but also teaches children about teamwork, discipline, and the value of practice.

4. **Martial Arts:** Classes in karate, judo, or taekwondo offer disciplined physical activity while instilling confidence and self-defense skills.

5. **Skating or Skateboarding:** Whether on ice in the winter or on pavement during warmer months, skating and skateboarding challenge balance, coordination, and endurance.

6. **Geocaching or Treasure Hunts:** This modern-day treasure hunting game uses GPS to find hidden items, encouraging children to walk, climb, and search in various terrains.

7. **Gardening:** Involving children in gardening tasks such as digging, planting, and weeding provides a gentle workout and teaches them about where food comes from.

8. **Animal Walks:** Encourage kids to imitate animal movements—hop like a frog, walk like a crab, or gallop like a horse. This playful form of exercise improves flexibility and strength in a fun, imaginative way.

9. **Rock Climbing:** Indoor rock-climbing gyms offer a safe environment for children to challenge themselves, build strength, and learn problem-solving skills.

10. **Family Fitness Challenges:** Create a family challenge that might include who can do the most push-ups, run a certain distance the fastest, or complete a mini-triathlon. Offering small rewards can motivate participation and healthy competition.

Incorporating these activities into a child's routine not only diversifies their physical exercise but also enriches their experiences and skills. From the teamwork learned in sports to the self-reliance taught in martial arts, each activity offers unique benefits that contribute to a child's overall development. Encouraging a broad spectrum of activities ensures that children find personal enjoyment in physical exercise, laying the foundation for a lifelong habit of staying active and healthy.

## Cool Down and Reflection:

After the workout, take a few minutes for a cool-down period. Lead the kids through some gentle stretches and deep breathing exercises to help them relax and reduce muscle tension. Then, gather in a circle for a quick reflection. Ask each child to share one thing they enjoyed about the workout and one thing they want to improve on next time.

It's clear that the secret to cultivating a love for physical activity in children lies in creativity, variety, and fun. This chapter has journeyed through a spectrum of engaging workouts specifically designed for the young ones, from playful warm-up activities and dynamic circuit training to imaginative obstacle courses and the calming practices of yoga. Each activity is tailored to turn exercise from a chore into an exciting adventure, fostering not just physical strength and agility but also a joyous engagement with movement.

Emphasizing the importance of fun in physical activity encourages children to view exercise not as a task but as a desirable part of their daily routine. The strategies outlined—leveraging the great outdoors for adventure, transforming chores into games, and throwing dance parties—underscore the myriad ways we can integrate exercise into children's lives in a manner that excites and inspires them. Moreover, involving children in the decision-making process of choosing activities empowers them and caters to their natural curiosity and need for autonomy.

Ultimately, the goal of these workouts goes beyond the immediate benefits of improved fitness and health; it's about laying the foundation for a lifelong appreciation for being active. By broadening children's horizons now, we not only enhance their current well-being but also equip them with the habits and mindset to lead healthy, active lives in the future.

# CHAPTER 12

## Breaking the Cycle of Bad Eating Habits: *A Parent's Guide*

As a parent, you play a crucial role in shaping your child's relationship with food and establishing healthy eating habits that will last a lifetime. Breaking the cycle of bad eating habits requires patience, persistence, and a proactive approach. In this chapter, we'll explore practical strategies to help guide your children toward healthier eating habits and set them up for long-term success.

**1. Lead by Example**: Children learn by example, so it's essential to model healthy eating behaviors yourself. Be mindful of your own food choices and attitudes toward food and demonstrate the importance of balanced nutrition in your daily life. Incorporate plenty of fruits, vegetables, whole grains, lean proteins, and healthy fats into your meals, and prioritize home-cooked meals over fast food or processed options. Research shows that children of parents who model healthy eating behaviors are more likely to develop similar habits. A study published in the International Journal of Behavioral Nutrition and Physical Activity found that parental role modeling was significantly associated with children's fruit and vegetable intake.

Strategies to effectively lead by example and model healthy eating behaviors for your children:

- **Practice mindful eating:**
  - Eat slowly and savor your food
  - Pay attention to hunger and fullness cues
  - Avoid distractions like phones or TV during meals
  - Discuss the flavors, textures, and nutritional benefits of foods during meals

- **Prepare and eat meals together:**
  - Involve children in meal planning and preparation
  - Have regular family meals where everyone eats the same foods
  - Use this time to model proper portion sizes and balanced meal composition

- **Verbalize positive attitudes about healthy foods:**
  - Express enthusiasm for fruits, vegetables, and other nutritious options
  - Avoid negative comments about foods you don't like
  - Frame healthy eating as enjoyable rather than a chore

- **Make nutritious snack choices visible:**
  - Keep a bowl of fresh fruit on the counter
  - Prepare cut vegetables and keep them at eye level in the refrigerator

- Choose healthy snacks for yourself when children are present

- **Demonstrate variety in your diet:**

  - Try new foods and recipes regularly

  - Include a diverse range of fruits, vegetables, whole grains, and proteins in your meals

  - Show willingness to retry foods you previously disliked

- **Practice moderation, not restriction:**

  - Allow yourself occasional treats in reasonable portions

  - Avoid labeling foods as "good" or "bad"

  - Demonstrate balance by including treats as part of an overall healthy diet

- **Prioritize home cooking:**

  - Plan meals in advance to avoid last-minute fast-food decisions

  - Batch cook healthy meals for busy days

  - Involve children in the cooking process to teach valuable skills

- **Show enthusiasm for healthy food shopping:**

  - Take children grocery shopping and model excitement about choosing fresh, nutritious foods

  - Teach them how to select ripe fruits and vegetables

- Discuss the nutritional benefits of different foods while shopping

- **Model healthy habits beyond just food choices:**

  - Stay hydrated by drinking water throughout the day

  - Engage in regular physical activity and invite children to join you

  - Practice stress-management techniques like deep breathing or meditation

- **Be consistent:**

  - Maintain healthy eating habits even when children aren't present

  - Avoid "hiding" unhealthy eating behaviors

  - If you make a less healthy choice, use it as a teaching moment of balance and moderation

- **Share your thought process:**

  - Verbalize why you're choosing certain foods or portions

  - Explain how different foods make you feel (energized, satisfied, etc.)

  - Discuss how your food choices align with your health goals

- **Handle setbacks positively:**

  - If you overeat or make an unhealthy choice, model a balanced response

- Avoid negative self-talk or extreme compensatory behaviors

- Demonstrate how to get back on track with the next meal or snack

**2. Create a Positive Food Environment**: Make your home a place where healthy eating is encouraged and celebrated. Keep a variety of nutritious foods readily available and limit the presence of unhealthy snacks and treats. Involve your children in meal planning and grocery shopping and let them choose healthy options that appeal to them. Create a relaxed and enjoyable atmosphere during mealtimes, free from pressure or conflict around food. Tip: Implement the "division of responsibility" approach developed by registered dietitian Ellyn Satter. Parents are responsible for what, when, and where food is served, while children are responsible for how much and whether they eat. This approach can reduce mealtime stress and promote healthier eating habits.

Strategies to create a positive food environment in your home:

- **Organize your kitchen for healthy choices:**

  - Keep nutritious foods at eye level in the refrigerator and pantry

  - Use clear containers to store pre-cut fruits and vegetables

  - Place healthier snacks in easily accessible locations

  - Store less healthy items out of sight or in hard-to-reach places

  - Use a fruit bowl as a centerpiece on the dining table

- **Implement a "taste adventure" system:**

  - Create a chart or board where family members can track new foods they've tried

  - Offer small rewards for trying a certain number of new healthy foods

  - Have themed meal nights featuring cuisines from different cultures

  - Encourage children to rate new foods on a fun scale (e.g., "yummy", "okay", "not for me yet")

  - Celebrate curiosity and openness to new flavors, rather than focusing on whether they liked the food

- **Establish positive mealtime rituals:**

  - Start meals with a moment of gratitude for the food

  - Create a pleasant ambiance with appropriate lighting and perhaps soft background music

  - Use special placemats or dishes for family meals to make them feel more special

  - Implement a "no negative food talk" rule during meals

  - Encourage conversation about topics other than food during mealtimes

- **Involve children in food-related activities:**

  - Assign age-appropriate tasks for meal preparation

  - Create a family cookbook with favorite healthy recipes

- Start a small herb or vegetable garden together

- Have children create weekly meal plans within certain nutritional guidelines

- Let children be "head chef" for one meal a week, guiding them towards healthy choices

- **Practice the division of responsibility consistently:**

  - Clearly communicate the parent and child roles in feeding

  - Provide structured meal and snack times

  - Offer a variety of foods at each meal, including at least one item you know your child likes

  - Avoid pressuring children to eat certain foods or clean their plates

  - Model enjoyment of a variety of foods yourself

  - Trust your child's appetite and allow them to stop eating when full

  - Avoid using food as a reward or punishment

**3. Educate and Empower**: Teach your children about the importance of nutrition and how different foods nourish their bodies and minds. Help them understand the difference between "everyday" foods that provide essential nutrients and "sometimes" foods that are okay to enjoy in moderation. Empower them to make informed choices about their food intake and encourage them to listen to their bodies' hunger and fullness cues. Activity: Create a "food rainbow" chart with your children, categorizing fruits and vegetables by color. Encourage

C.R. PURZ

them to eat a variety of colors each day to ensure they're getting a wide range of nutrients.

**4. Set Clear Boundaries**: While it's important to allow flexibility and occasional treats, establish clear boundaries around food choices to prevent overindulgence and promote balance. Discuss the concept of moderation with your children and establish guidelines for how often and how much they can enjoy sweets, snacks, and unhealthy foods. Stick to consistent meal and snack times to help regulate hunger and prevent mindless eating. A study published in the journal Appetite found that children whose parents set consistent limits on food intake had better self-regulation skills and were less likely to overeat.

**5. Encourage Variety and Adventure**: Introduce your children to a wide range of foods from an early age and encourage them to explore new flavors, textures, and cuisines. Make mealtime an adventure by trying new recipes together, experimenting with different ingredients, and involving your children in cooking and food preparation. Emphasize the importance of variety and balance in their diet to ensure they receive a wide array of nutrients. Implement the "one bite rule" - encourage children to try at least one bite of a new food, but don't force them to finish it if they don't like it. It can take up to 15-20 exposures to a new food before a child accepts it.

**6. Promote Positive Body Image**: Foster a healthy body image in your children by focusing on their overall health and well-being rather than their weight or appearance. Encourage them to listen to their bodies and trust their internal cues rather than external influences. Avoid labeling foods as "good" or "bad" and instead emphasize the importance of nourishing their bodies with wholesome foods that make them feel good. A study published in the International Journal

- 110 -

of Eating Disorders found that parental comments about weight and eating habits were significantly associated with disordered eating behaviors in children.

Strategies to promote positive body image in children:

- **Focus on health and functionality over appearance:**
  - Emphasize what bodies can do rather than how they look
  - Celebrate physical achievements (e.g., learning a new skill, improving endurance)
  - Discuss how different foods nourish the body and support various functions
  - Avoid commenting on your own or others' weight or body shape

- **Encourage body respect and acceptance:**
  - Teach children that bodies come in all shapes and sizes
  - Help them identify and appreciate their unique physical traits
  - Promote self-care practices like proper hygiene, sleep, and physical activity
  - Discourage negative self-talk and model positive self-acceptance

- **Develop media literacy skills:**
  - Discuss unrealistic body standards in media with your children

- Teach them to critically analyze advertisements and social media content

- Encourage them to follow diverse role models who promote body positivity

- Limit exposure to media that promotes unhealthy body ideals

- **Reframe language around food and eating:**

  - Avoid labeling foods as "good" or "bad"

  - Use neutral terms like "everyday foods" and "sometimes foods"

  - Discuss foods in terms of how they make the body feel (energized, strong, focused)

  - Encourage a balanced approach to eating that includes all food groups

  - Talk about "fuel" for the body rather than calories or fat content

  - Emphasize enjoyment and variety in eating rather than restriction or control

- **Create a body-positive home environment:**

  - Remove scales from visible areas or consider not having one at all

  - Avoid negative talk about your own or others' bodies

  - Compliment children on non-appearance related qualities (e.g., kindness, creativity)

- Foster open communication about body image concerns and offer support

**7. Be Patient and Supportive**: Changing eating habits takes time, so be patient and supportive as your children navigate this journey. Offer praise and encouragement for their efforts and celebrate their successes along the way. Be prepared for setbacks and challenges and approach them with empathy and understanding rather than criticism or punishment. Remember that your goal is to help your children develop a healthy and positive relationship with food that will serve them well throughout their lives.

**8. Address Emotional Eating**: Help your children develop healthy coping mechanisms for dealing with emotions instead of turning to food for comfort. Teach them to identify and express their feelings and provide alternative ways to manage stress or boredom. Create an "emotion toolbox" with your child, filled with activities they can do when feeling upset, such as drawing, listening to music, or practicing deep breathing exercises.

Strategies to address emotional eating in children:

- **Teach emotional awareness and expression:**
  - Help children identify and name their emotions
  - Use emotion charts or cards to visualize different feelings
  - Encourage regular "feeling check-ins" throughout the day
  - Model expressing your own emotions in healthy ways

- Practice active listening when children share their feelings

- **Create an "emotion toolbox":**
  - Work with your child to identify calming activities they enjoy
  - Include items like coloring books, stress balls, or fidget toys
  - Add cards with simple breathing exercises or mindfulness prompts
  - Include a list of physical activities like jumping jacks or dancing
  - Regularly update the toolbox to maintain interest and effectiveness

- **Develop alternative coping strategies:**
  - Teach simple meditation or mindfulness techniques
  - Practice deep breathing exercises together
  - Encourage journaling or drawing to express feelings
  - Introduce age-appropriate problem-solving techniques
  - Engage in physical activities as a way to process emotions

- **Foster a supportive environment:**
  - Create regular opportunities for open communication

- Validate your child's feelings without judgment

- Avoid using food as a reward or comfort

- Encourage seeking support from trusted adults or friends

- Model healthy ways of dealing with stress and emotions

- **Establish a routine for emotional check-ins:**

   - Set up regular "emotion talk" times, such as during car rides or before bed

   - Create a daily or weekly family sharing circle where everyone discusses their feelings

   - Use a mood tracker or journal to help children monitor their emotions over time

   - Implement a "feelings thermometer" to help kids gauge the intensity of their emotions

   - Develop a family ritual for processing difficult emotions together, like a weekly "worry dump" session

**9. Limit Screen Time During Meals**: Encourage mindful eating by turning off screens during mealtimes. This allows for better family communication and helps children focus on their food, leading to improved satiety cues and potentially reduced overeating. A study published in Pediatrics found that children who watched TV during family meals consumed fewer fruits and vegetables and more pizza, snack foods, and sodas than those who didn't.

Strategies to limit screen time during meals and promote mindful eating:

- **Establish a "no screens at the table" rule:**
    - Create a designated area for devices during mealtimes
    - Turn off or silence phones, tablets, and TVs
    - Make this rule apply to all family members, including adults
    - Explain the importance of this rule to children in age-appropriate terms

- **Create engaging mealtime alternatives:**
    - Use conversation starter cards or games to encourage discussion
    - Share highlights of your day or play "high-low" (best and worst parts of the day)
    - Tell stories or jokes to keep the atmosphere light and fun
    - For younger children, use colorful placemats with educational content or games

- **Practice mindful eating techniques:**
    - Encourage everyone to take a few deep breaths before eating
    - Teach children to observe their food using all senses before eating

- ◦ Discuss the flavors, textures, and origins of the foods on the plate

- ◦ Encourage slower eating by putting utensils down between bites

- **Make mealtimes a family bonding opportunity:**

  - ◦ Involve children in meal preparation and table setting

  - ◦ Use meals as a time to plan future family activities

  - ◦ Create special theme nights (e.g., "Taco Tuesday" or "Breakfast for Dinner")

  - ◦ Rotate responsibility for choosing dinner topics or activities

- **Gradually reduce screen dependence:**

  - ◦ If cold turkey is too difficult, start by having one or two screen-free meals per week

  - ◦ Gradually increase the number of screen-free meals

  - ◦ For resistant family members, set a timer for a short period of screen-free eating, then gradually increase the time

**10. Teach Nutrition Label Reading**: As children get older, teach them how to read and understand nutrition labels. This skill will empower them to make informed choices about their food intake, even when you're not around to guide them. Turn grocery shopping into a scavenger hunt, challenging your children to find foods that meet certain nutritional criteria (e.g., high in fiber, low in added sugars).

This chapter has illuminated a path forward for parents seeking to guide their children away from the pitfalls of unhealthy eating patterns toward a relationship with food that is balanced, nutritious, and joyful. Through leading by example, creating a positive food environment, educating and empowering children, setting clear boundaries, encouraging variety, promoting positive body image, and providing patient and supportive guidance, parents can lay the groundwork for their children's long-term health and well-being.

Embracing these strategies, parents can transform mealtime from a potential battleground into an opportunity for growth, discovery, and connection. By fostering an atmosphere where healthy choices are not only accessible but also appealing, we can encourage children to explore and enjoy the richness of a well-rounded diet. The journey to break the cycle of bad eating habits is not one that will be completed overnight, but with each small step, we move closer to instilling in our children the values of mindful eating and self-care.

Remember, the goal is not perfection but progress. Every positive change, no matter how small, is a step towards a healthier future for your child. Stay committed, be consistent, and celebrate the journey towards better eating habits as a family.

# CHAPTER 13

## Fortifying Our Children Against the Onslaught of Unhealthy Food Marketing

---

In today's digital age, children are bombarded with sophisticated marketing strategies aimed at promoting processed foods, candies, and sodas. These advertisements are meticulously designed to captivate the young mind, making the task of protecting our children a daunting yet vital undertaking. The mission to safeguard our youth from these persuasive tactics necessitates a holistic and proactive approach, intertwining education, policy intervention, community engagement, and personal responsibility.

## Building Robust Media Literacy

A cornerstone in defending children against the seduction of unhealthy food marketing is the development of robust media literacy. By educating our children on the mechanics behind advertisements and the persuasive techniques employed by marketers, we empower them with the ability to critically analyze and question the content they encounter. Interactive workshops and school programs that simulate advertising scenarios can be instrumental in teaching children to recognize and deconstruct marketing gimmicks, fostering an environment of informed skepticism.

## Nurturing a Positive Food Culture

Counteracting the allure of processed foods requires the cultivation of a positive food culture within homes and communities. This involves not only making nutritious foods accessible but also celebrating the joy of healthy eating through family traditions, community farmers' markets, and school gardening programs. By elevating the status of whole foods and creating positive associations with healthy eating, we can diminish the desirability of unhealthy alternatives.

## Setting Boundaries Around Screen Exposure

With the digital realm being a primary avenue for food marketers, regulating screen time emerges as a critical strategy in reducing children's exposure to such advertisements. Implementing structured screen time schedules, coupled with engaging children in discussions about the content they view, can significantly mitigate the impact of advertising. Encouraging alternative pastimes that promote physical activity and personal interaction offers a healthy counterbalance to screen consumption.

## Championing Policy Advocacy and Reform

To effect systemic change, concerted efforts in policy advocacy and reform are essential. This includes rallying for legislation that restricts the marketing of unhealthy food products in children's media and public spaces. Supporting initiatives that mandate clear, truthful labeling of food products can also aid in this battle, enabling caregivers and children alike to make informed food choices. Policy changes, however, require the voice and support of the community to be realized, highlighting the importance of collective action and advocacy.

## Engaging in Community-Wide Education

Educating the broader community about the effects of unhealthy food marketing on children's health is paramount. Through seminars, public campaigns, and social media, communities can raise awareness about the importance of protecting our children from manipulative food advertisements. Schools, in partnership with health professionals and local businesses, can spearhead these educational initiatives, creating a unified front against the marketing of unhealthy foods.

## Modeling Healthy Lifestyles

Ultimately, the battle against unhealthy food marketing is deeply personal, with parents and caregivers at the forefront. By embodying healthy lifestyle choices and demonstrating the value of nutrition and physical well-being, adults set a powerful example for children. Sharing experiences, such as cooking healthy meals together or participating in physical activities, can instill lifelong habits that prioritize health and well-being over the fleeting allure of processed foods.

The battle against the pervasive influence of processed food advertising is multifaceted and complex. Yet, with the right tools, strategies, and community support, it is a battle that can be won. This chapter underscores the critical need for a holistic approach that encompasses media literacy, a nurturing food culture, mindful screen time management, advocacy for policy reform, and, fundamentally, the modeling of healthy lifestyle choices by parents and caregivers.

Educating our children to become discerning viewers, capable of critically assessing the marketing messages bombarding them daily, equips them with a vital shield against manipulation. By intertwining this media literacy with the cultivation of a positive relationship with food, we can counteract the allure of unhealthy options and instill a preference for nutritious choices. Moreover, engaging in policy advocacy and community education amplifies our collective voice, pushing for systemic changes that safeguard our children's health and well-being.

Ultimately, the responsibility of guiding our children through this commercialized landscape rests with each of us. Through deliberate actions, conversations, and choices, we can illuminate the path to a healthier future for our children.

# CHAPTER 14

## Summary: *The Impact of Processed Foods and Sugars on Children's Health*

---

The consumption of processed foods, refined sugars, fructose, and added sugars is a growing concern, particularly in the context of children's health and development. The allure of convenience and taste masks the underlying risks these foods pose, ranging from obesity and metabolic disorders to behavioral changes and nutritional deficiencies.

- **Obesity and Metabolic Disorders:** The link between processed foods, high sugar intake, and obesity is well-documented. These foods, often calorie-dense yet nutritionally void, contribute to excessive weight gain and related conditions such as type 2 diabetes. The mechanism often involves insulin resistance and an imbalance in energy dynamics.

- **Dental Problems:** Sugar's role in dental health deterioration cannot be overstated. Consumed in large amounts, it fuels bacteria in the mouth that produce acids, attacking the tooth enamel and leading to cavities and decay.

- **Behavioral and Cognitive Effects:** The impact of diet on behavior and cognitive development is profound. Foods high in sugar can cause significant fluctuations in blood sugar levels, leading to hyperactivity, concentration difficulties, and mood swings. Over time, this can affect a child's academic performance and social interactions, underscoring the need for dietary vigilance.

- **Nutritional Deficiencies:** A diet high in processed foods often comes at the expense of whole foods, leading to a lack of essential nutrients. This can hinder growth, compromise immune function, and affect overall health, making it crucial to prioritize nutrient-dense foods.

To counteract these negative effects, a multifaceted strategy is essential:

1. **Education and Awareness:** Teaching children about healthy eating and the importance of nutrient-dense foods over processed options can empower them to make better food choices.
   REF: https://pubmed.ncbi.nlm.nih.gov/30280308/

2. **Incorporate Whole Foods:** Shifting focus to whole foods such as fruits, vegetables, lean proteins, and whole grains can provide the necessary nutrients for children's growth and development without the adverse effects of processed foods and added sugars.
   REF: https://pubmed.ncbi.nlm.nih.gov/17243492/

3. **Healthy Snacking:** Replacing sugary or highly processed snacks with healthier alternatives like fresh fruits or

vegetable sticks with hummus can satisfy hunger in a nutritious manner.

https://pubmed.ncbi.nlm.nih.gov/17243492/

4. **Cooking Together:** Engaging children in meal preparation not only teaches them valuable skills but also fosters a healthy relationship with food. Home-cooked meals allow for better control over ingredients and encourage a move away from reliance on processed foods.

5. **Moderation and Balance:** Understanding that an occasional treat is acceptable can help children learn about moderation and balance, aiding them in making healthier choices without feeling restricted.

6. **Lead by Example:** Children often mimic adult behaviors, including eating habits. By modeling healthy eating, adults can significantly influence their children's dietary choices and attitudes towards nutrition.

Addressing the challenge of processed foods and sugars in children's diets requires a holistic approach that values nutrition education, whole foods, and the cultivation of a positive food culture. By embracing these principles, it is possible to safeguard children's health, supporting their physical, cognitive, and emotional well-being on the journey towards a healthier future.

Concluding Chapter 14, "The Impact of Processed Foods and Sugars on Children's Health," underscores a critical health concern that extends beyond the dining table into every aspect of a child's life. This chapter has painted a comprehensive picture of how processed foods and added sugars detrimentally affect children's physical health, contributing to obesity, metabolic disorders, dental problems, and nutritional deficiencies. Moreover, it has shed light on the less visible, yet equally concerning, repercussions on behavioral and cognitive development, highlighting the stark link between diet and a child's ability to learn, concentrate, and interact socially.

Amid these challenges, the chapter also offers a beacon of hope, outlining actionable strategies for reversing these trends. Through education and awareness, prioritizing whole foods, fostering healthy snacking habits, engaging children in cooking, and modeling balanced eating behaviors, parents and caregivers can steer children away from the pitfalls of processed foods. It emphasizes that the journey toward healthier eating is not about prohibition but about making informed, mindful choices that celebrate the richness and variety of nutritious foods.

The role of parents and caregivers is pivotal in this endeavor. By leading by example and creating an environment where whole, nutrient-dense foods are the norm rather than the exception, we can instill in our children the values of good nutrition and the skills to make healthy dietary choices. This chapter serves not just as a guide but as a call to action for all who influence children's dietary habits. Together, we can break the cycle of reliance on processed foods and open up a new path—a path that leads to enhanced health, vitality, and well-being for our children, setting the stage for a lifetime of positive eating habits and a deep-rooted appreciation for the power of nourishment.

REF: https://pubmed.ncbi.nlm.nih.gov/28921869/
https://pubmed.ncbi.nlm.nih.gov/27550974/
https://pubmed.ncbi.nlm.nih.gov/34836143/

# THE SUPERFOODS SQUAD: *OPERATION NUTRI-POWER*

## Chapter 1: A Mysterious Energy Crisis

In the bustling city of Nutriopolis, something strange is happening people are feeling tired and sluggish, unable to enjoy their usual activities. A group of friends, known as the Superfoods Squad, sets out to investigate. These are not ordinary friends; they're nutrients come to life, each with special powers based on their health benefits.

- **Challenge**: Identify foods in your kitchen that are high in vitamins and minerals. What superpowers might they have?

## Chapter 2: Captain Carrot's Vision Quest

First up is Captain Carrot, rich in beta-carotene, which the body converts into vitamin A, essential for good vision and immune function. Captain Carrot leads a mission to help the citizens of Nutriopolis see the importance of including vitamin-rich foods in their diets.

- **Experiment**: Try eating a carrot snack and reading in different lighting conditions. Does it make a difference in how well you see?

# Chapter 3: The Hydration Operation with Aqua-Melon

Aqua-Melon, with her ability to control water, teaches the squad about the importance of hydration for maintaining energy levels and keeping the body functioning properly. She demonstrates how even mild dehydration can lead to fatigue and decreased focus.

- **Activity**: Track your water intake for a day. Do you notice a difference in how you feel when you're well-hydrated?

# Chapter 4: Spinach Ninja and the Muscle Mystery

Spinach Ninja, packed with iron and magnesium, shows how these minerals support muscle function and energy production. The squad faces a challenge that requires physical strength, and Spinach Ninja's nutrients are key to their success.

- **Workout Challenge**: Create a simple exercise routine. Observe how your strength and stamina improve with regular physical activity and a nutrient-rich diet.

# Chapter 5: The Sweet Science with Fruity Duo

The Fruity Duo, Apple and Berry, tackle the misconception that all sugars are bad. They explain the difference between natural sugars in fruit, which come with vitamins, fiber, and water, and added sugars, which can lead to energy crashes.

- **Science Activity**: Compare the labels of various snacks. Which ones have natural sugars and which have added sugars?

## Chapter 6: Broccoli Bro and the Immune System Invasion

Broccoli Bro dives into how antioxidants and vitamins in green vegetables can strengthen the immune system. When a wave of colds hits Nutriopolis, Broccoli Bro's nutrients help shield the city's inhabitants from getting sick.

- **Immune Boost Plan**: Design a colorful, nutrient-packed meal plan for a week that includes a variety of fruits and vegetables.

## Chapter 7: Epic Showdown: Balance vs. Binge

The Superfoods Squad faces their ultimate test against the Junk Food Juggernauts in a battle of balance versus binge. They learn that while it's okay to enjoy treats in moderation, relying on them can lead to energy crashes and health problems.

- **Debate**: Have a debate with friends or family about the role of balance in diet. Can you have your cake and eat it too, healthily?

## Epilogue: Heroes of Nutriopolis

The Superfoods Squad's adventures teach the kids of Nutriopolis that eating a balanced diet, staying hydrated, and exercising are all key to becoming everyday heroes in their own lives. They learn that making informed choices about their health can give them the energy to pursue their dreams.

- **Project**: Create a Superfoods Squad comic strip based on your own healthy eating adventure. What challenge does your squad face, and how do they overcome it?

# GLOSSARY

- **Processed Foods:** Foods that have been altered from their natural state for convenience, shelf life, or taste. They often contain additives, preservatives, and artificial flavors.

- **Added Sugars:** Sugars and sweeteners added to foods and drinks during processing or preparation. This includes ingredients like high-fructose corn syrup and white sugar.

- **Fructose:** A type of simple sugar found naturally in fruit, honey, and vegetables, but also used as an added sugar in many processed foods and beverages.

- **Obesity:** A medical condition characterized by excessive body fat that increases the risk of health problems such as type 2 diabetes, heart disease, and certain cancers.

- **Metabolic Disorders:** Health conditions that disrupt normal metabolism, the process by which your body converts food into energy. These can include diabetes, obesity, and metabolic syndrome.

- **Dental Problems:** Health issues affecting the teeth and gums, often caused by sugary foods and drinks which promote tooth decay and cavities.

- **Behavioral and Cognitive Effects:** Changes in behavior or brain function, such as difficulty concentrating or mood swings, often linked to diet and nutritional intake.

- **Nutritional Deficiencies:** Conditions caused by not getting enough of the essential nutrients needed for good health, which can affect growth, immune function, and overall well-being.

- **Whole Foods:** Foods that are minimally processed and as close to their natural form as possible, including fruits, vegetables, whole grains, nuts, and seeds.

- **Healthy Snacking:** Eating snacks that are nutritious and beneficial to health, as opposed to snacks high in sugars, fats, and calories with little nutritional value.

- **Moderation and Balance:** The practice of consuming foods in moderate amounts within a varied and balanced diet to maintain good health.

- **High-Fructose Corn Syrup (HFCS):** A sweetener made from corn starch that has been processed to convert its glucose into fructose. It is commonly found in many processed foods and beverages due to its sweetness and low cost.

- **Insulin Resistance:** A condition in which the body's cells become less responsive to the hormone insulin, which regulates blood sugar levels. It can lead to increased blood sugar levels and is a risk factor for developing type 2 diabetes.

- **Type 2 Diabetes:** A chronic condition that affects the way the body processes blood sugar (glucose). It is characterized by high blood sugar, insulin resistance, and a relative lack of insulin.

- **Metabolic Syndrome:** A cluster of conditions that occur together, increasing the risk of heart disease, stroke, and type 2 diabetes. These conditions include increased blood pressure, high blood sugar, excess body fat around the waist, and abnormal cholesterol levels.

- **Non-Alcoholic Fatty Liver Disease (NAFLD)\*\*:** A range of liver conditions affecting people who drink little to no alcohol. It's marked by the accumulation of fat in the liver, leading to inflammation and potential liver damage.

- **Dental Erosion:** The loss of tooth enamel caused by acidic foods and drinks. This can lead to cavities and other dental issues.

- **Hyperactivity:** A condition characterized by excessive movement, impulsiveness, and difficulty paying attention. Diet, particularly high sugar intake, can influence hyperactive behavior in some children.

- **Leptin:** A hormone involved in regulating energy balance by inhibiting hunger, which in turn diminishes fat storage in adipocytes (fat cells).

- **Gut Microbiome:** The complex community of microorganisms living in the digestive tracts of humans and other animals. Diet significantly influences the composition of the gut microbiome, which in turn can affect overall health.

- **Probiotics**: Live bacteria and yeasts that are beneficial for health, especially the digestive system. They are often referred to as "good" or "helpful" bacteria because they help keep the gut healthy.

- **Whole Grain:** Refers to grains that have all three parts of the grain kernel (the bran, germ, and endosperm) in their original proportions. Whole grains are more nutritious and provide more fiber, vitamins, and minerals than refined grains.

- **Refined Sugars:** Sugars and syrups that are added to foods or beverages during processing or preparation. They are also found in sugary drinks and most processed foods and can contribute to various health issues when consumed in excess.

- **Nutrient-Dense Foods:** Foods that have a high nutrient content relative to their calorie content. These foods contain vitamins, minerals, complex carbohydrates, lean protein, and healthy fats.

- **Empty Calories:** Calories from foods and drinks that contain little to no nutrients. These often come from sugars and fats found in processed and fast foods.

- **Food Labeling:** The information about a food item's ingredients and nutritional content on its packaging, which can help consumers make informed choices about their food purchases.